Recovering from Depression

III

Recovering from Depression

Answers to Common Questions

Lesli Kramer, M.D.

SYREN BOOK COMPANY
Saint Paul

Most Syren Book Company books are available at special quantity discounts for bulk purchases for sales promotions, premiums, fund-raising, and educational needs. For details, write Syren Book Company, Special Sales Department, 2402 University Avenue West, Suite 206, Saint Paul, Minnesota 55114.

Published by
Syren Book Company LLC
2402 University Avenue West
Saint Paul, Minnesota 55114

Cover design: Kyle G. Hunter
Cover photo: Lesli Kramer

Printed in the United States of America on acid-free paper.

ISBN 0-929636-23-6

LCCN 2004102300

To order additional copies of this book see the order form at the back of the book or Amazon.com

*This book is dedicated to the many people
I have met over the years who have said,
"If you ever want someone to provide
a testimonial, I'll be happy to do it."
This book is part of your testimonial,
and a tribute to all of the people who
have taken the necessary leap of faith
to feel better.*

Table of Contents

help? • What should I expect from my doctor? What might my doctor expect of me? • What medication should I take? Which one is the best? • How exactly do antidepressants work? • What can I expect when I start taking medication? Do I need to worry about side effects? • How long will it take before I feel better? • What if the medication isn't working? • What are some of the first signs of improvement? • How will I know that I'm getting better? • What if I feel better, but not completely better? • What if I have been taking medication and doing well, then start to feel bad? • Do medications cure depression? • Can I cut back on my dosage once I feel better? • How long should I take medication? • What should I consider if I am going to stop the medication? Can I stop medication on my own? • What are the chances of having another episode? • Phototherapy • Electroconvulsive Therapy (ECT) • Are "natural" treatments safe and effective? • Are herbal preparations chemically active? • There are potential dangers in treating yourself

• Try to keep a regular routine • Try to have a balanced diet • Try to develop healthy sleep habits • Avoid alcohol and drugs • Try to exercise • Try to overcome inertia • Accomplish tasks by setting reasonable goals • Limit the quantity of work that you set out to do • Limit the amount of time you spend on a task • Give yourself credit for your accomplishments • Plan your day • Allow yourself the opportunity to do things for enjoyment—make time for play and relaxation • Chip away at social isolation • Habits • Stay in the present • Don't look too far ahead • Avoid getting stuck in the past • Avoid negative experiences • Place emphasis on things that go right (rather than things that go wrong) • Try not to make major decisions • Don't drive if you are distracted

• Certain thought patterns and behaviors increase stress • Try to worry less about what other people think • It is okay to say NO • Anger and conflict resolution • Avoiding conflict and "stuffing" anger can be a problem • Assertiveness • Try to discuss your anger when you have calmed down • Some ways to have a fair argument • You don't have to be perfect (none of us are) • Practice healthy detachment; let go of things you can't control • Feel your own feelings • Try to avoid guilt, shame, and blame • Work on letting go of little things • Driving recklessly is an unhealthy emotional release • Work on recognizing when you are feeling overwhelmed • Avoid avoidance • Time management

Foreword

If you have depression, you probably have some questions about what that means and what can be done about it. The prospect of seeking help can be overwhelming and people often stop before they even get started. Taking the first steps toward getting help can be easier and less intimidating if you begin with some basic information.

This book provides an introductory-level overview of depression, written with the hope that you will feel encouraged about the potential for recovering from this treatable disorder. It addresses some of the most common questions and concerns people express in the beginning stages of treatment, topics that are often discussed when a person first meets with a doctor. This is an affirming, reassuring book for those who are suffering or recovering from depression, and it provides helpful information for family members, friends, and other concerned individuals.

Information is presented in a brief format, allowing you to learn about depression without being overwhelmed by details. In-depth theoretical discussions about the underlying mechanisms of depression are beyond the intended scope of this book and are not included. General issues with regard to medication treatment are covered but information about specific medications and their side effects has been excluded. The content centers on depression and does not go into detail about related conditions, such as bipolar disorder (manic-depressive illness). Reading this book is a first step in learning about depression. If you discover that you want to learn more, there are many fine books that provide comprehensive details. A list of additional resources can be found at the end of this book.

There are seven main subject areas addressed in this book: general information about depression, medical treatment of depression, psychotherapy, self-help strategies, ideas for decreasing susceptibility to depression, the impact of depression on family members and friends, and suggestions for helping the person with depression. Each subject area is divided into short topics that can be read one at a time. The table of contents lists all of the topics covered in each section, allowing you to easily find items of interest.

Recovering from Depression

/ / /

General Information about Depression

A few words about stigma

The stigma associated with depression, including the fear of being labeled as "mentally ill" or "crazy," prevents many people from seeking help. Derogatory terms abound in our culture, all of which feed into misperceptions and stereotypes. Depression is a brain syndrome, no less valid than other brain illnesses such as Parkinson's disease and multiple sclerosis. Those afflicted with depression or other brain illnesses are not "crazy." People sometimes think that depression is their fault, but it is a medical condition, just as diabetes, high blood pressure, and cancer are real physical problems. None of these illnesses are caused by personal weakness. No one is to blame.

A sense of shame and feeling "different" from other people can add to the burden of having depression. If you have depression, rest assured that you are not alone. Countless people throughout the ages, in every culture and country in the world, have suffered from depression. Millions of people in the United States have depression now, and about one in five Americans experience a depressive episode at some point in their life.

Since depression does not necessarily entail symptoms that the casual observer might notice, people who are unfamiliar with it sometimes have difficulty understanding that it is a medical problem. Though depression may not be readily apparent, it is not less real than any other illness. People with diabetes or high blood pressure do not have external manifestations of their illness, yet the validity of those conditions is not called into question. Depression is a physical condition too. Once upon a time, many people erroneously believed that doing something underhanded or sinful brought on cancer. Today, few people would ever consider that a person's character caused their cancer. Hopefully someday the same will hold true for people with depression.

The media conveys mixed attitudes about depression, reflecting the attitudes of society at large. On one hand, there is some excellent educational coverage with well-balanced and up-to-date presentations. On the other hand, depression is sometimes used as material for jokes and "entertainment." People often joke about topics that are uncomfortable, but jokes about depression trivialize a serious illness. Depression isn't funny. We don't generally poke fun at people with diabetes or cancer, yet it is often still "open season" on people who take medications for depression. People with depression are not inherently lazy, stupid, weak, or deranged. They are people with an illness, which can be mild or severe. They may be rich or poor, young or old. They are normal people from all walks of life.

It is not unusual to hear people remark that we are an overmedicated society, turning to pills for trivial reasons or to solve all of our problems. Some popular magazines and television shows have promoted that notion, using this type of "headline" to grab the attention of potential readers or viewers. Repeated exposure to misleading "sound bites" can impact public perception of an issue. Sometimes the content of these articles or shows actually debunks the "headline," but the damage is already done because many people never get beyond the hype.

Treating depression is not the same as popping a pill for recreational purposes. However, untreated depression is the culprit behind a lot of alcohol and drug abuse. Comments suggesting that people simply need to develop better coping skills reflect a lack of understanding about the nature of depression and do a disservice to those individuals who are directly impacted by it.

People who experience their first episode of depression frequently report that they had no idea that it could be so overwhelming. Until a person has experienced depression up close and personal, it can be hard to understand how completely and utterly it can rip apart the fabric of a person's life. Ideal treatment of depression involves a comprehensive approach that includes psychotherapy and common-sense strategies for good self-care in addition to medications.

Unfortunately, the majority of people who have depression do not seek treatment. Untreated depression is the cause of much unnecessary suffering, disability and death. Depression may contribute to mortality from other physical problems, such as heart attacks. People may become apathetic and find it difficult to take care of themselves or turn to unhealthy behavior, such as smoking, overeating and the abuse of drugs and alcohol, as a method of coping with depression. Some people with depression cause their deaths directly, through suicide. Most people with depression do not really want to die; they want to get better, but they have lost hope and can't stand the thought of going through the rest of their lives feeling miserable. Even relatively mild depression can adversely affect a person's productivity, relationships with friends and family, and general state of health. Depression, regardless of its severity, can be treated successfully. There is hope. The challenge is to convey hope to the person with depression.

What is Depression?

The term "depression" is confusing since people often say that they are "depressed" when they feel bad about something. Everyone feels down, discouraged, unhappy, or "depressed" at times. "Depression" is not the same as normal sadness or grief. It doesn't even necessarily involve feeling sad about something that has happened, though it can sometimes be triggered by stressful events.

Depression is a syndrome, with both physical and emotional symptoms, that occurs when there have been changes in the balance of different chemical systems in the brain. Just as the symptoms of the common cold are caused by a number of different viruses, the specific chemical problem in depression may vary from person to person or family to family. The brain is a complex organ that is very difficult to study directly. Much is still unknown about the biology of depression, but our knowledge is expanding rapidly.

A person's brain is the command center of their entire body. The brain receives, filters, stores, and sends out information via electrochemical and chemical means. The brain secretes chemicals that regulate the function of other organs, such as the thyroid and adrenal glands, which in turn secrete chemicals that impact brain function. The brain regulates many processes, including sleep cycles, appetite, energy level, mood, motivation, sexual interest, pain sensation, memory, and concentration. When brain chemistry is out of balance, some or all of these areas can be affected.

Symptoms such as disturbed sleep or increased need for sleep, fatigue, depressed mood, anger or irritability, anxiety, excessive worry, and restlessness are common. Problems with concentration and memory can interfere with school or work performance or the ability to function at home. It can be difficult to start and follow through on tasks. One person with depression may feel profoundly sad while the next might feel emotionally flat or numb, with a sense of emptiness. There can be loss of enjoyment during activities that are normally pleasurable and people lose interest in their pastimes. Self-confidence and self-esteem are often affected. There may be an increase or decrease in appetite. People may pay less attention to their physical appearance. Sexual interest can evaporate. Some people may feel consumed by guilt.

People may lose hope that they will ever feel good again and suicidal thoughts can occur. If you or someone you know has suicidal thoughts, you should seek help now. Everything may feel hopeless to the person with depression, but it is not hopeless. You or the person you care about can feel better.

The physical components of depression often overshadow the emotional components. General fatigue and malaise, headaches, muscular aches and pains, gastrointestinal problems, and a host of other symptoms are common in depression. These are real symptoms, caused by depression. People can feel so physically ill that they worry that their symptoms may be caused by cancer or a brain tumor. Depression is one of the most common conditions seen in a primary-care doctor's office. People see their doctor because they feel physically ill and may have no idea that depression is the cause of their symptoms. Even if they do suspect depression, people often hope that some other "physical" cause can be found because they equate depression with a failing of personal fortitude. People need to be aware that depression *is* a physical problem and is not caused by personal shortcomings.

Recognition of depression can be a challenge; even doctors sometimes have a hard time identifying it. People suffering from depression do not always have identical symptoms. Life experiences, environment, personality styles, genetic and physical makeup vary from person to person, and these factors can influence the form depression takes in each individual. The symptoms can also change over time, and people may not realize that they are all a part of the same process. Depression can begin suddenly but more often it comes on gradually. Mild depression can be difficult to detect, especially when it has been present for a long time, because people do not remember, or perhaps never knew, what it feels like to be free from symptoms.

The recognition of depression is further complicated because there are other conditions that have symptoms that overlap and sometimes coexist with depression. In children, behavioral changes or school problems may dominate the picture. They may be diagnosed with attention deficit disorder. In older people, the problems with concentration and memory that can occur in depression may be confused with Alzheimer's disease. It is important not to miss the diagnosis of depression in these situations because appropriate treatment can lead to significant improvement.

What causes depression?

At present, there is no tidy answer to this question. It is likely that the syndrome identified as depression is a cluster of similar appearing conditions caused by a variety of different alterations in brain chemistry. There are many different brain circuits and chemicals that interact in complicated ways and a slight change at any point in one of these pathways could cause a problem with the entire system. As an analogy, consider a traffic jam. An accident, poor road conditions, malfunctioning traffic lights, or a slow driver could cause traffic to back up. There can be many possible explanations but the result is the same. Now consider your brain. It is vastly more complicated, similar to linking all the roadways from every major city in the world.

Previous theories that speculated that depression stemmed *entirely* from things such as unresolved childhood issues, learned helplessness, or anger turned inwards are no longer widely held beliefs. These theories were narrowly focused and did not factor in the complex relationships between physical and emotional stresses, environment, psychological reactions, biology, and genetic predisposition. Many factors can influence a person's vulnerability to the development of depression, such as abuse, the traumatic loss of a parent in childhood, divorce, bereavement, serious illness, financial difficulties, legal problems, occupational or school problems, or other stresses encountered in daily life. It is not unusual for people with a family history of depression to manifest symptoms for the first time after a psychological stress or physical event, such as illness, puberty, or childbirth. For some people, however, it is an inherited disorder that can "just happen," without any apparent external trigger.

Many people are unaware that depression runs in their family because it is not talked about openly and it may not be outwardly obvious to others. Some family members may have very severe depression that is difficult to hide, while others, who are not as severely affected, may be able to put up a good front. Even without a family history, it is possible for people to develop depression if subjected to enough psychological or physical stress. No one can claim complete invulnerability.

Certain medical conditions, such as strokes, Parkinson's disease, heart attacks, and multiple sclerosis are associated with an increased risk of depression. This depression is not merely a "psychological" reaction to having a bad thing happen, but a real biological change induced by the initial condition.

What if it is not depression?
What if it is something else?

Some illnesses can first manifest with depressive symptoms. Diabetes, lupus, hypothyroidism (low thyroid hormone), anemia, and vitamin B_{12} deficiency are just a few examples of disorders that can cause symptoms that mimic depression. If one of these conditions is responsible for the depression, it is important to identify and treat the primary disorder.

Depression can be caused by a number of different medications, such as steroids or certain high blood pressure medications. Alcohol or drugs may cause depressive symptoms. If you are taking a medication known to cause depression, your doctor may need to discontinue it or find an alternative. Elderly people may be especially sensitive to medications and interactions between medications, since their bodies are no longer able to process drugs as efficiently as when they were younger and their brains may be more vulnerable to side effects. It is important for a doctor to evaluate all the medications a person is taking and to consider possible side effects and interactions.

Even though other illnesses can occasionally masquerade as depression and should be considered among the diagnostic possibilities, it is equally important not to put depression at the bottom of the list of potential culprits. A lot of time can be wasted chasing down laboratory test after laboratory test, trying to look for rare causes of depressive symptoms. Other disorders often have unique physical symptoms (or clusters of symptoms) that can be identified when you discuss your situation with a doctor. Depending upon your individual symptoms and history, your doctor may want to check some blood tests and/or administer a thorough physical exam.

What role does stress play in depression?

"Stress" is not a precise term, but it is a term that most of us use to describe the negative emotional and physical impact of events that we perceive as overwhelming or threatening. Stress is not the same from person to person. Events that are stressful to one person may be exhilarating to the next. Sometimes if a stressor is predictable it is easier to mentally prepare for it, whereas it may be perceived as more stressful if it occurs out of the blue. The degree to which a person feels they have control over the stressful situation can also affect the perception of feeling stressed. If a person can identify that they have options, they may not feel as stressed. Additionally, if a person can recognize those things beyond their control, it is sometimes easier to let go and not worry as much.

As an example of stress affecting physical functioning, consider stepping off a curb and nearly being hit by a car. You would probably experience heart racing, rapid breathing, and shakiness. Nothing physically touched you, but the automatic fear response affected your body. Likewise, other types of stress can affect the way your body works. A single stressful event or the accumulation of a lot of different stresses can produce physical changes that precipitate depression. Sometimes even "good" stress, such as a desired move or job change, can upset the body's balance and trigger depression. People who have gotten through stressful times in the past without difficulty might find themselves worn down and less resilient when exposed to chronic or repeated stress. Depression can be triggered by a relatively minor event, similar to the proverbial "straw that broke the camel's back." This often takes people by surprise because they realize their response to the small stress is out of proportion to the event. Even people who are generally able to handle nearly anything can develop depression. If a person already has depression, stressful events can make it worse.

But I don't have any reason to be depressed

Depression *can* happen without any apparent cause. The depression could be a biological change that is caused by something internal we simply are not able to pinpoint. People often try to identify why they are depressed, but there may be no external reason. Depression is a condition, an alteration in brain function that can "just happen." A person who had their initial episode of depression triggered by stress can later develop a pattern in which the onset of depression does not have any close correlation with life events. A person can develop depression even when everything in their life seems good from the outside. People often find some source of stress in their life and use that to explain their depression; it is human nature to look outside ourselves for cause and effect, but there may be no connection.

Is depression normal during bereavement?

Depressive symptoms, such as loss of appetite or inability to sleep, are very common when a person has experienced a significant loss, and are generally short-term. Feelings of extreme guilt, lowered self-esteem, a sense of worthlessness or hopelessness, and suicidal thoughts are often present in depression but are not commonly part of a typical grief process. Bereavement is a significant stress, however, and can trigger an actual depressive episode. Treating depression in the context of bereavement does not "cover up" the grief. Depression often shuts down feelings or the ability to process feelings, and treating it can allow one to proceed through the grief process more normally.

What if I only have premenstrual depressive symptoms?

Hormonal changes can impact the way our brains function. There are significant hormonal fluctuations premenstrually, postpartum, and preceding menopause, and some women may be susceptible to depressive symptoms at these times. The fluctuating levels of hormones likely impact other brain chemicals. Not every woman with mild premenstrual mood changes has depression; in fact, most women do not. "Premenstrual dysphoric disorder (PMDD)" is the current term used for more severe premenstrual symptoms (formerly termed premenstrual syndrome or PMS). If there are symptoms that interfere with a woman's ability to function or adversely impact relationships, they bear a closer look.

In addition, many women with depression experience a significant worsening of their depressive symptoms premenstrually. Some women may notice more prominent symptoms of anxiety and irritability rather than feeling depressed. A woman with a mild depressive disorder or depression that is only partially treated may feel fairly good during the first two or three weeks of her menstrual cycle, only to slip back down into depression in the week or two before her menstrual period. This is an indication that the depression is not yet fully under control. Depressive symptoms, whether premenstrual or present throughout the entire month, can be successfully treated.

Some people take offense at and express concern about "labeling" women with premenstrual symptoms, thus making a "disorder" out of "normal" monthly fluctuations. Consider the situation in which a woman has a thyroid disorder triggered by changes associated with pregnancy. We don't pretend that the thyroid disorder is normal, even if it was triggered by a "normal" event in a woman's life (pregnancy). We diagnose and treat it. The more we shy away from simply dealing with the depression or PMDD that some women experience, the more we give credence to stigma. It would be more fruitful to work on decreasing the stigma of depression and emphasizing recognition and treatment for the women who do have a depressive disorder. Pretending that depression does not exist sends a message that it's not real, that it's "all in her head" and that she should just snap out of it. Again, not every woman has depression or premenstrual dysphoric disorder, but if she does, it should be taken seriously. While jokes about PMS abound, depression and premenstrual dysphoric disorder are not a laughing matter for the women affected.

What about pregnancy and postpartum depression?

It was once thought that pregnancy protected women from depression, but we now know that this is not true. Women with a history of depression also have a higher risk of developing depression in the postpartum period. Many women go through mood changes or "baby blues" that are temporary and resolve on their own. If, however, the mood changes do not resolve within a couple of weeks, are severe, or interfere with a woman's ability to function, it is advisable to seek a psychiatric consultation. The months after birth are both precious and stressful. Depression robs a new mother of joy and an extended illness can interfere with bonding and the ability to care for the baby.

Depression is not a benign condition for women and their babies, either during pregnancy or after the baby is born. Psychotherapy is often helpful and there are now medications available that many women have used safely during pregnancy and breastfeeding. Many obstetricians are comfortable with prescribing antidepressant medications but if they do not want to initiate treatment themselves, they should be able to provide the name of a psychiatrist to turn to for evaluation. It is important to have access to information about the potential risks and benefits associated with treatment as well as information about the risks associated with *not* treating depression. If a medication is prescribed, it is essential to have regular follow-up to ensure that the depression is fully treated. Early treatment and full recovery helps the whole family get off to a better start.

A rare but even more serious situation is postpartum psychosis (a depression accompanied by delusions and/or hallucinations), which may place both the mother and child at risk. Confusion and extreme agitation are cause for concern. If a woman has developed postpartum psychosis, it is critical to obtain treatment as soon as possible.

If you are pregnant, tell your obstetrician about any previous episodes of depression you have experienced and let your doctor know if you develop symptoms during or after your pregnancy.

I don't feel depressed. How can it be depression?

Unfortunately, the term "depression" does not accurately describe the disorder. It is possible to have depression and not even feel "depressed" or sad. Your mood may be flat, you may not enjoy activities like you did in the past, or you might find that you are completely unable to experience pleasure. You might be anxious or worried, fearful or irritable. The major manifestation can be feeling physically ill. You may know that you feel awful, but have no idea what is wrong. People often see their doctors for these physical symptoms without knowing that depression could be the root of their problems. Fatigue, insomnia, headaches, stomach problems, nausea, dizziness, and generalized aches and pains can all be manifestations of depression. The actual problem may not be recognized because the symptoms can fool you or your doctor into thinking that something else is going on. When people have prominent physical problems, they often assume that their anxiety or depressed mood is simply a natural consequence of being worried about their health, and they do not always recognize that their emotional state and physical symptoms are part of the same process.

If you have a number of unexplained symptoms, depression should be considered early on, before too much time passes. People sometimes undergo numerous tests to try to identify a "physical problem" and then find out that the tests were normal and that "nothing is wrong." There may not be anything wrong with those tests, but something is wrong or you wouldn't be going to a doctor in the first place. Without a proper diagnosis, you may begin to wonder if it is all "in your head" or worry that other people will think that you are a hypochondriac. These symptoms are real; you are not imagining them. Receiving a correct diagnosis and finally having an explanation for your symptoms can be a relief and a first step in the process of getting better.

Is it normal to be depressed in the context of a serious health problem?

Feeling sad or down at times is expected, but it is not normal to have depression. There are many instances

GENERAL INFORMATION ABOUT DEPRESSION

in which depression is overlooked because the symptoms seem fitting under the circumstances. For example, when someone is suffering from a significant illness such as cancer, the possibility of coexisting depression is not always considered. It is normal to experience some depressive symptoms in these situations, such as fatigue and feelings of sadness, but if the symptoms are severe, do not resolve, or interfere with life's daily activities, a professional consultation should be considered. It is easy to rationalize that the way you are feeling is normal, even if you are feeling very bad. Not everyone with a serious medical illness will develop depression, but for those who do, treatment can help. When the depression is treated, people often discover that they can still find enjoyment and satisfaction in their lives. They have less of a tendency to "give up" or retreat from their lives and loved ones. Even people with a mild depressive disorder can benefit from treatment. Treating the depression can help people deal with their other illness more effectively.

Is it possible to stop depression by relieving stress?

Finding ways to manage the stressors in your life is very helpful, but when the stress subsides, depression may not automatically lift; a person does not always

22 | LESLI KRAMER, M.D.

"bounce back" once the stress is alleviated. As an analogy, consider the situation in which you have stayed out in the sun too long. Coming in out of the sun is helpful, but you still have to deal with a painful burn. Once depression has begun, it can have a life of its own. You may not realize that the depression is or has become a separate problem until the stress goes away. Having depression can also make you more sensitive to stress, just like being sunburned makes you more sensitive to the sun.

How is depression diagnosed?

At this point in time there is not a blood test or brain scan that can be used to diagnose depression. The chemical changes in the brain that are associated with depression are not reflected as measurable changes in the chemical composition of the bloodstream, and are consequently not detected by blood tests. New brain scan technology is making it possible to learn more about brain functioning, but we are not at the point where these scans can be used to provide a definitive diagnosis of depression. Many people feel uncomfortable because of the lack of conclusive tools to aid in the diagnostic process. Technology permeates our lives, yet the brain is still a vastly uncharted territory. More is known about brain functioning today than ever before, but there is still much to understand. Someday there may be tests to "confirm" a diagnosis of depression, but keep in mind that the most important part of the evaluation for any illness is usually the discussion you have with your doctor about your symptoms. Many illnesses, including depression, are diagnosed primarily on the basis of the history you give to your doctor.

Medical Treatment of Depression

Treatment with medications: general issues

There *are* effective treatments for depression. It is possible to feel good again. Antidepressant medications are now a mainstay in the treatment of depression. Your chances for recovering from depression are almost always greater if you include antidepressant medication as one of the ways you take care of yourself. You do not have to feel miserable and endure depression indefinitely.

One note of caution must be made with regard to reading other people's personal accounts of their experience with depression. People rarely feel compelled to write about treatment that was highly successful. They are too busy living their lives. Stories about "good outcomes" are also less likely to catch other people's attention because it is simply less interesting to read about uncomplicated recovery than it is to read about a monumental struggle. Hence, reading about personal experiences can leave you with a sense of futility and a skewed impression that treatment rarely provides substantial benefit. Not everyone has a perfect outcome, but in the vast majority of situations medication can alleviate the symptoms of depression.

In the past, there were not as many options for medical treatment. Older medications frequently caused side effects that were difficult to tolerate. Increasing knowledge about the balance and interaction of chemical systems in the brain has made it possible to develop medications that specifically target these systems, which in turn leads to fewer undesirable side effects. There are now many medication choices available, and the side effects are generally more tolerable.

Medications are not a "quick fix" for depression but for many people they are enormously beneficial. As with many other illnesses, engaging in healthy activities and approaching treatment in a comprehensive manner will generally lead to a more successful outcome. Someone with diabetes will have better control of their illness if they watch their diet, exercise, monitor blood sugar carefully, and take their insulin. Someone with high blood pressure may benefit from exercising and losing weight as well as taking a medication. All of these measures contribute to better health. In depression, medications may be a central part of treatment, but many people also benefit from talk therapy. Getting exercise, eating well-balanced meals, and avoiding alcohol and drugs are other important ways to take care of yourself.

Many people are reluctant to take medication, for a variety of reasons. Some people do not like medications, period. Others fear feeling drugged or emotionally numbed. People worry that they will not "be themselves" or that they will develop dependence on a medication. People are concerned about side effects. These are all normal concerns. Talking to a doctor can help you obtain the information you need about what you can expect from a medication.

Many people don't seek help until they feel like they have "hit a wall." Things finally get so bad that something has to change. As terrible as it is to get to this point, it can also be the beginning of hope for the future.

How will a medication make me feel?

When you are treated with a medication for depression, you should feel like yourself, but like yourself on a decent day. Not drugged and not euphorically happy, but simply like yourself. Depression can make you feel emotionally numb, angry, anxious, or depressed out of proportion to the situation. When your depression is fully treated, your normal range of emotional reactions should be restored. If you do not feel like yourself again, or if your emotions feel blunted, your depression has not been successfully treated.

Do medications mask problems?

Medication doesn't make you feel constantly happy. It isn't a crutch. It doesn't make you forget the problems in your life. Once the medication has treated the depression, however, you should regain the capacity for experiencing happiness and be able to handle the problems in your life more easily. You may find that some things you thought were important had been blown out of proportion, but you will still be able to recognize real problems. The difference is that it may be easier cope with problems or do something about them. When people are treated for depression, they often become less complacent and less likely to put up with unhealthy situations; they are better able to recognize problems that were masked by the depression and need to be dealt with. It may be easier to identify and work on changing behavior patterns that feed into depression.

Will medications change my personality?

This is a complicated question. Undoubtedly, a person who has had depression all of their life has been shaped to some extent by the experience of depression. A person's personality structure is generally relatively stable by the time they become an adult. However, depression may accentuate underlying personality characteristics, making them more prominent than they would normally be. An example of this might be a tendency to be passive, pessimistic, or cantankerous. A person may also have characteristics that are not apparent until the depression is treated, such as a good sense of humor. Depression can act as a mask, and treating it can be like lifting a shroud and revealing what is hidden. People experiencing their first depression typically report that they do not feel like themselves during the episode. When the depression is treated, they report that they feel like they are back to their normal self again. People who have always had depression (or who have had it a long time) may have a more difficult time knowing what their normal personality would be like, in the absence of depression. For these individuals, recovering from depression can be a gratifying process of discovery.

Do medications shut down creativity?

While some artists have produced great works during a depression, many find their creativity shut down. It is usually difficult to produce much of anything while depressed. The wellspring of ideas, the spark, is generally lacking and there is no energy to be productive. For the most part, writers can't write, painters can't paint, and composers can't compose when they are suffering from depression. When their depression is lifted, most people find that their creativity has been set free.

The relationship between creativity and depression has often been romanticized and we are drawn to the tragic stories of artists who have led agonized lives. There has been great debate over the years about the notion that artists are especially prone to depression, but scant evidence exists for this hypothesis.

The experience of depression can undoubtedly shape the *direction* of artistic expression. Any experience, including the inner turmoil of depression, can influence an artist. Anyone who has suffered with depression can understand its painful depths, but artists are able to translate and express their internal experiences through their own particular art form.

At times it has been suggested that perhaps artists are more prone to depression because they are introspective and more attuned to serious contemplation of the human condition whereas other people live their lives with blinders on. However, it is important to consider that depression can act as a filter, shifting and often constricting a person's perceptions and range of emotions. The world is viewed through the lens of depression. Once depression has lifted, there may actually be a greater appreciation of the range of human experience. Living in the depths of depression is not a prerequisite for creative expression.

Are antidepressants addictive? Will they make me feel intoxicated or impaired?

Antidepressant medications are not addictive. They do not make you feel high and they don't cause any sort of craving. Antidepressant medications are not "happy pills" and they don't make people without depression feel better than normal. It would be like taking a blood pressure medicine if you don't have high blood pressure; it is not going to give you better than normal blood pressure. Taking an antidepressant medication is similar to taking insulin or a thyroid supplement. You are not addicted to it; your body simply needs it in order to be healthy and stay in the right chemical balance.

I don't like to take pills. Can't I just tough it out?

Many people don't like the idea of any sort of medication. They often avoid medications for headaches or other common ailments, preferring to "tough it out" until the problem goes away. Unfortunately, with depression and other major illnesses, waiting it out doesn't work very well. Most of the time, the illness isn't going to resolve itself quickly, if ever, and it can last a long time. If you have high blood pressure and leave it untreated, it can lead to a number of cardiovascular problems. Untreated diabetes can cause problems with vision, circulation, nerve and kidney function. Over time, untreated depression can lead to serious problems. Waiting for depression to go away on its own may mean feeling bad for an extended period of time and running the risk of complications in all areas of your life: work, school, family, and relationships in general. Depression can rob you of quality time. Depression can get worse and become more difficult to treat. Over time, depression may be harmful to the areas of your brain involved in memory and other cognitive processes. Depression can be bad for your overall health; you may not take care of yourself the way you should and the changes in your brain chemistry can negatively impact other parts of your body.

How can one little pill make a difference?

One pill *can* make a difference. With many other medical problems, such as high blood pressure, heart disease, thyroid disease, vitamin deficiencies, and hormonal imbalances, small chemical changes can make a huge difference. The same is true for depression.

Maybe it will just get better on its own

Depression can fool you; some days may be better than others, causing you to think it's improving. One day slips into the next, but when you look back, you realize there have been more bad days than there should have been. Other illnesses can also have that same kind of day-to-day variability. Someone with high blood pressure may have a good blood pressure reading one day and a bad one the next. People often put off treatment, hoping that it will get better on its own. If you think you might have depression, rather than delaying any longer, consider setting up a consultation with a doctor who has experience in diagnosing depression. While it is possible to have a spontaneous remission from depression, it may take a long time or may never occur. Depression, left untreated, can get worse, become more persistent, and alter the course of your life.

Should I be able to deal with it by myself?

People sometimes think that if they need to take medication, it is a failure on their part or a sign of weakness. They think that they should be able to "deal with it" on their own. Many people do try to deal with it for a long time, often working very hard in therapy, eating healthy foods, exercising, and doing other things to try to take care of themselves. If there were any way to get rid of it on their own, through sheer willpower, they surely would have done just that. People don't want to feel depressed, but you can no more wish away depression than you could wish away a stroke, Alzheimer's disease, or multiple sclerosis. If you had diabetes and had to take insulin to stay healthy, doing so would not be a sign of weakness. Taking medication for depression is not a sign of failure, but instead it is one of the ways you can take care of yourself. Taking charge and taking care of yourself is a sign of strength.

Can I work it out in therapy?

Treatment with medication can help people with depression make more productive use of therapy. Depression can muddle a person's thought processes, making it difficult to make progress in therapy. In the past, it was not unusual for therapists to consider referring their patients for a medication evaluation only as a last resort. With a wider understanding of the biological implications of depression, therapists often prefer that a patient be treated with medications early on in the process of therapy. Without treatment, therapy can get bogged down and go around in circles. With treatment, a person's thought processes become more coherent and the important issues for psychotherapy can be clarified. As you feel better, you can work in therapy to make changes or resolve issues that will eventually culminate in you feeling even better.

Some specific therapies, such as interpersonal and cognitive behavioral therapy, have been shown to be helpful in the treatment of depression. For patients with severe depression, medication alone is more effective than psychotherapy alone, but a combined approach is most beneficial. If you have had depression for many years, even if it has not been severe, psychotherapy should be strongly considered as part of you treatment program. In general, medication works faster and more reliably across a broader range of people than psychotherapy, but for many people a skilled therapist can be worth their weight in gold.

Who can help?

A first step in the treatment process is often a visit to your primary-care doctor. Many family practitioners and internal medicine specialists treat depression,

but if your physician does not feel like your treatment
falls within his or her area of expertise, you might be
referred to a psychiatrist. It is also reasonable to work
with a psychiatrist from the beginning, since they are
medical doctors who specialize in the treatment of
depression as well as other brain disorders that result
in emotional, physical, and behavioral changes. You
can ask your family doctor, friends, a medical society,
local university, or mental health support organization
for the names of psychiatrists in your area. There are
many ways to start the process of finding help; the
important thing is to take that first step.

It is important to have a physician who is well
trained in the diagnosis and treatment of depression.
Your doctor needs to be able to differentiate between
depression and other illnesses that mimic depression. It is also essential to screen for bipolar disorder
(manic-depressive illness) because the treatment strat-
egy is different. Bipolar disorder involves both periods
of depression and episodes of mania or hypomania (a
less dramatic form of mania). Symptoms such as un-
usually rapid speech, racing thoughts, euphoria, irritability, rapidly changing moods, higher than normal
energy, a decreased need for sleep, increased impul-
sivity, sudden creativity or grandiose plans are common during the manic or hypomanic component of
bipolar disorder. It is extremely important to identify
these types of symptoms, even if they occurred in the

distant past, because treatment with antidepressants alone can make bipolar disorder worse. A person who is currently experiencing depression may not remember these past episodes, or consider them to be pertinent history, so it is important that your doctor asks about them.

If your primary-care doctor has tried a couple of different medications without success, it makes sense to see a psychiatrist. If you have complicating factors such as substance abuse, serious relationship problems, a family history of bipolar disorder, suicidal thoughts, delusions, and/or hallucinations (uncommon but possible with severe depression), you should see a psychiatrist.

There is often confusion about the difference between a psychiatrist and a psychologist. A psychiatrist is a physician who can prescribe medication and has had training in psychotherapy (counseling). A psychologist has specialized training in psychotherapy, and some also perform psychological testing. A psychologist attends graduate school and can attain a doctorate in psychology (a Ph.D. or Psy.D.) whereas a psychiatrist is an M.D. who has attended medical school followed by an internship then a residency program focusing on psychiatry. Social workers, psychologists, psychiatric nurses, and psychiatrists all can function as "psychotherapists." A psychiatrist might focus on the medical aspects of treating depression and refer you to a different person for psychotherapy, or a psychiatrist might be involved in both the management of medication and psychotherapy.

What should I expect from my doctor?
What might my doctor expect of me?

In order for you to receive the best and most appropriate care, you will need to thoroughly and honestly discuss your symptoms with your doctor. This is not the time to hold things back or try to present yourself in the best possible light. For example, you should talk to your doctor if you think that you may have a problem with an eating disorder, gambling, money, sexuality, alcohol, or drugs. Your doctor is there to help you, not to make judgments. Your doctor should listen to your concerns, answer your questions, and provide information about treatment options and what to expect, including side effects and how long it might take to feel better.

You should feel like you are listened to and treated respectfully at all times and that the relationship with your doctor is collaborative. It is important for you to feel like you can develop a trusting relationship with your doctor. You should feel like the atmosphere is open and that your questions are welcomed. Don't hesitate to ask questions, and if you don't understand something, ask for clarification. Sometimes it takes a couple of sessions to have a sense for whether it will be a good match for you. If the doctor doesn't seem like a good fit, consider seeking a consultation with another. Even competent doctors are not a perfect fit for every person.

During the first session, which is generally longer than follow-up sessions, your doctor will want to obtain a complete history from you, including all physical and emotional symptoms, a review of all current medications, and your medical and family history. It is helpful to discuss any stress that you are under and the ways in which the depression is affecting your life. Your doctor might recommend some laboratory tests to rule out certain other illnesses that might be confused with depression, but laboratory testing is not necessarily indicated in every situation. Your doctor will give you an opinion and recommendations for treatment. Last, but not least, your doctor should provide hope.

It is important to have follow-up sessions with your doctor in order to evaluate whether or not the medication is working at the prescribed dose, review side effects, and discuss any questions you may have about your treatment. Treatment for other conditions, such as high blood pressure or elevated cholesterol, requires periodic assessment; the same holds true for the treatment of depression. If you are given a prescription for an antidepressant, make certain to schedule an appointment for reassessment of the medication within about four to six weeks, or sooner if necessary.

What medication should I take?
Which one is the best?

No one antidepressant is necessarily "the best" medication. Since there may be a variety of different problems with brain chemistry and function that can result in depression, medications with different chemical mechanisms may work in different people. A medication may work well for one person but not for the next. One person may not have any side effects while the next person experiences every side effect in the book. Everyone has a different physical make-up.

There is no way to determine ahead of time which medication will be right for you, but there are a number of things to consider. The choice of medication may be influenced by coexistent illnesses or other medications you are taking. If a family member has had a good response to a medication, your doctor might consider starting with it; while not everyone will react in an identical fashion, a medication that is effective for one family member may be effective for another. Another important consideration is the dosing schedule, especially because it is often difficult to remember to take something more than once daily. Any medication, including antidepressants, can have side effects and those side effects could be beneficial or unwanted. Talking to a doctor can help you sort through the advantages and disadvantages associated with the different medication choices.

How exactly do antidepressants work?

The theories and details of what is known about the chemical basis of depression lie beyond the scope of this book, but we do know that three major brain chemicals (also known as neurotransmitters) affected by our current medications are dopamine, norepinephrine, and serotonin. Neurotransmitters facilitate communication between brain cells (neurons) and regulate their activity. Neurotransmitters released by one brain cell can attach to other brain cells by latching onto a receptor that fits their shape and chemistry (like fitting together two pieces in a puzzle). Antidepressants can elevate the levels of these naturally occurring neurotransmitters and affect the activity of receptors. Your brain uses these chemicals to regulate activity in brain pathways similar to the way you use your brake pedal or accelerator to respond to changes in traffic flow. You can speed up to go around a slow moving vehicle or slam on the brakes to avoid hitting a piece of debris in the roadway. You may not know why the other vehicle is moving slowly or how the debris came to be on the road, but you can respond. Likewise, the underlying causes of depression are unknown, but changing the levels of regulatory neurotransmitters can alleviate the symptoms.

We cannot determine what brain pathways or chemicals might be most critical in a given individual and there is currently no clinical test that can answer that question for us. If this notion makes you uncomfortable, and it's understandable if it does, bear in mind that much of the medical field has had to operate in this fashion. We generally know that things work and what the side effects are before we know why they work. Aspirin has long been known to treat aches and pains, but we didn't know how it worked. We now have much more information about its mechanism of action, but it hasn't changed the way we use the medication for pain in any significant fashion. Using the knowledge we have, to the best of our abilities, even if we don't know all the answers, is a fact of life when it comes to the field of medicine.

What can I expect when I start taking medication? Do I need to worry about side effects?

A lower-than-normal dose is often used when a medication is first prescribed. Starting low and, as necessary, gradually increasing the dosage allows your body time to get used to it. It is possible to feel worse temporarily after beginning a medication because side effects usually occur early on in treatment, whereas the benefit may not be apparent for several weeks. You may not have any problems with side effects, but if you do, they frequently improve in a couple of weeks. It is important to let your doctor know if you are having problems. If you experience troublesome side effects, your doctor may lower your dosage or recommend other things to help you feel more comfortable as you adjust to the medication. The side effects of newer medications tend to be bothersome or annoying rather than medically serious, but keep in mind that you get to make the final decision about whether a side effect is intolerable or whether you can tough it out. On occasion there are "media scares" that present concerns about various medications, including antidepressants. It is always prudent to examine these concerns fully by turning to professionals with the expertise to answer your questions.

How long will it take before I feel better?

Waiting is difficult, but antidepressant medications do not work right away for most people. For some, improvement may start within a few days or after a week or so. For most people, however, the benefits don't show up for two to four weeks, or sometimes longer. Improvement can sometimes happen so gradually that you don't realize you're feeling better until you stop and really think about how you were feeling previously.

Treatment for many medical problems can take time to become effective. It pays off to stick with the process. You need to take the medication on a daily basis and you need to keep taking it. If you don't feel better after four to six weeks, as long as you are not having any major problems with side effects, your doctor will probably recommend that you increase the dosage of your medication.

The most common reasons for treatment failure are not taking the medication long enough, not taking it regularly, or not being on a sufficient dose for your body. It is important to have a doctor who pursues treatment in a diligent, rational manner rather than rapidly switching from one medication to the next. People sometimes think that "if a medication hasn't worked by now" it's not going to work at all, but if your dose isn't at the right level for your body, it simply can't work. You may need a higher dose. If you had a headache and only bit off a tiny piece of an aspirin, it probably wouldn't help a lot. The same concept applies to antidepressant treatment. A dosage that is just right for one person may be far too low for the next.

The severity of the depression doesn't really determine what dosage will be needed; an individual's physical and chemical make-up is the most important factor. If somebody doesn't absorb medications well or if their body is very efficient at getting rid of medications, a higher dose is needed just to get a normal level into their system. Body size can make a difference at times, though this is not always the most significant determining factor. Smoking, gender, and other medications can impact the level of antidepressant that is required. Thus, as a consequence of varying physical characteristics, it is possible for someone with mild depression to need a high dose and someone with severe depression to need only a low dose.

What if the medication isn't working?

The chances are good that you will respond to the antidepressant you start with, but don't give up hope if it doesn't work. You might simply need a different medication. There are many choices and one of them should work for you. On occasion, it can take several months to discover the correct medication or dosage, but it is important to remember that almost everyone can be successfully treated for depression. The key is to keep trying. Don't give up. Even people with chronic depression, who have taken a number of medications, can often finally find a medication that is right for them. New medications are being developed at an encouraging rate as well. Everyone is built a little differently and we need all the medication options we can get. We are not clones of one another and neither are the medications.

If it seems like you aren't getting better, talk to your doctor about it. Your doctor should scrutinize whether you have been prescribed a high enough dosage for a sufficient period of time. Also, keep in mind that it is quite common for people to forget pills, even if they are taken just once per day. People often take out their pill bottle, even open it, then walk away and don't remember whether or not they actually took the pill. Using a "pill reminder" container can be very helpful, even if you only take one pill. It's easy to simply open the lid for that day and check whether or not the pill is gone.

Your doctor may need to reconsider your diagnosis, check to see if something was missed, and review whether other medications, drugs, or alcohol are complicating the picture. If another illness is causing the depressive symptoms, there may not have been any other physical indication of the illness early on, except for the depression. As the illness progresses, other symptoms may become more evident. It is important to identify and treat those illnesses or the depressive symptoms will not lift.

What are some of the first signs of improvement?

As you start to get better, other people may notice a positive change before you actually start to feel better. There may be changes in the way you look and in the way you interact with others. That is not unusual. You may still feel lousy but the fact that you look better is a positive sign. Next you may feel better, even before your memory and ability to concentrate completely improve. (People often look better before they feel better and feel better before they think better.) Your level of depression can fluctuate from day to day, so you may have an up and down course as you are getting better. Try not to get discouraged if you have some bad days, but instead look for a general trend of improvement. If you have even one good day after not having any for a long time, that is a positive sign.

How will I know that I'm getting better?

People often wonder how they will be able to determine when the medication is working. If your depression is of recent onset, you will know when you feel better. You should feel like yourself again. If you have always had a low level of depression, it can be a little hard to know what to expect. While it can be difficult to convey in words what it is like to have the depression lift (just as it can be difficult to convey in words what the experience of depression feels like), some of the types of statements that people make speak for themselves . . .

- It was like a curtain lifting.
- I can laugh again. I have my sense of humor back.
- I used to feel irritated all the time. Now I'm so much more patient with my kids.
- I feel like I'm more grounded.
- It was like switching from black and white to color.
- I couldn't feel anything before. It was all flat and meaningless. Even my kids couldn't arouse any feeling in me. I am so thankful that I can feel again.
- My life hasn't changed, but it just seems easier to deal with things.
- I can take things in stride.
- It felt like I was in an ocean . . . I was drowning . . . waves of despair washed over me . . . now I'm finally on firm ground.

- I'm normally not a person who cries, but I kept finding myself in tears. Now I feel in control of my emotions instead of my emotions being in control of me.
- I feel like myself again.
- It was like a huge weight was lifted off my shoulders.
- I couldn't stand it. At the time I thought only death would bring me peace, but I really didn't want to die. Now I feel good and at peace again. The medication saved my life.
- I didn't have any reason to feel unhappy. I didn't know what was going on but it was awful. I never would have thought that what I had was depression. I'm so glad it was diagnosed and so glad that I am feeling better.
- It is so refreshing to look forward to things again.
- I don't think I realized how bad I felt until I started to feel better again.
- My thoughts would churn around and around, spinning endlessly. I didn't get anywhere with them. I can finally think something through and then let it go.

- I can make plans again, without having to wonder if I am going to feel well enough to follow through.
- It seems like I can see things so much more clearly. It was like the fog rolled out.
- I put off doing anything about it for years. I wish it hadn't taken me so long, but I'm glad that I finally did something.
- It's such a relief.
- It dawned on me that I'm finally feeling like I am supposed to feel.
- I feel like I got my life back.
- Somehow I got through it for all those years but I never want to have to do that again.

If a person has low-level depression simmering for years, they may not actually know they have it until the depression comes to a full boil. With treatment comes the realization that not only is the severe depression gone, but they actually feel better than they have felt for a long time. It is similar to walking around for years not knowing that you need glasses or a hearing aid. When you finally get them, you experience the world with a new clarity.

What if I feel better, but not completely better?

The goal of treatment should be full remission of symptoms, with complete restoration of previous health and ability to function. It is not enough to aim for only partial improvement or somewhat improved ability to function. Without a full remission, there is an increased risk of relapsing back into depression. The vast majority of people can feel completely better, so if you don't, talk to your doctor. Don't assume that you have to live with it.

What if I have been taking medication and doing well, then start to feel bad?

If you begin to slip back into depression, it may mean that the intensity of the underlying illness has increased and that the medication dosage you are taking is no longer enough. It could mean that other factors are feeding into the depression, such as increased stress or the use of alcohol. Perhaps you have become less vigilant about taking the medication on a regular basis. Occasionally people may develop tolerance to their medication. Even if that happens, however, it doesn't mean you are out of luck. Your doctor may be able to increase your dosage, add another medication, or switch to a different medication. There are a lot of options. You shouldn't try to adjust your medications on your own. Instead, call your doctor or make an appointment.

Do medications cure depression?

Antidepressants do not cure depression the way antibiotics cure an infection, but the medications do effectively treat it. The treatments for many illnesses, such as diabetes, hypothyroidism, high blood pressure, and high cholesterol, are aimed at restoring a normal chemical balance in the body and controlling the symptoms, rather than curing the actual underlying problem. The same thing applies to depression treatment. If you stop the medication and your illness is still active, you will redevelop your depressive symptoms.

Can I cut back on my dosage once I feel better?

It is important to stay on the dose of medication that helped bring you out of your depression. Most attempts to get by with a lower maintenance dose result in a return of depressive symptoms. Just as a person with high blood pressure needs a certain level of medication to keep their blood pressure stable, a person with depression needs to keep their medication at a therapeutic level.

How long should I take medication?

Your doctor can provide you with the information you need to be able to make this decision. In general, if this is your first or second episode of depression, the current recommendation is to take the medication for about one year. Long-term treatment should be considered after a third episode or when there has been a pattern of chronic depression (even if it is mild), as there is a high risk of redeveloping depression if medication is discontinued. If you have had severe suicidal thoughts, a serious suicide attempt, serious depression that was difficult to treat or depression accompanied by delusions and/or hallucinations, ongoing treatment may be considered even before a third episode of depression. Even if long-term treatment is recommended, it's important to remember that you are the one who gets to decide if you are going to continue on the medication, and you certainly don't have to make that decision ahead of time.

What should I consider if I am going to stop the medication? Can I stop medication on my own?

People are often tempted to stop taking medication on their own. When a person has felt good for a long time, it is not uncommon to question whether medication is still necessary. It may be difficult to remember how bad it felt when the depression was in full swing, and people wonder how they would feel without the medication. Rather than try to stop the medication on your own, it is wise to consult with your physician. These medications are not addictive, but you can have side effects, or your depression could return suddenly, if you stop some of them too abruptly. Your doctor is there to help you. Remember, you still get to make the final decision about whether you stay on a medication or not. Talking with your doctor can help you make an informed decision.

Timing can be an important consideration. If possible, don't stop taking your medication when there is a lot of stress in your life or right before a big event, even if it is a good event. More than a few vacations have been spoiled that way. If you have seasonal depression, wait until spring or summer to stop. There is no way, at present, to determine if the depression has resolved itself, so you and your doctor have to pick a time that seems reasonable and then just give it a try. You will generally taper down on the medication rather than stop it suddenly. Before you stop taking the medication, it is useful to review the symptoms you had toward the beginning of your depression, so you can be on the lookout for re-emerging problems. If you are going to redevelop symptoms, they may not show up immediately—it could be weeks or months down the line before they come back. If your symptoms do recur, it makes sense to consult your doctor and get started on the medication again.

What are the chances of having another episode?

Unfortunately, once depression has been triggered, there is a greater risk of experiencing another episode of depression in the future. We now recognize that depression is often a chronic or recurrent illness rather than a self-limited singular experience. More than half of the people who experience one episode of depression will experience a second episode. Once a person has had a third episode, the risk of recurrence is about ninety percent. The good news is that depression is treatable.

Phototherapy

In some people, depression is triggered by the change of seasons and decreasing length of day. This tendency is often accompanied by an increased appetite and need for sleep. You can conceptualize it as being akin to the biological trigger that tells a bear that it's time to hibernate. When you think about it, this tendency probably would have had great value as we were evolving. If you eat a lot, conserve energy by sleeping, and feel lethargic so you don't go outside where either a predator or inclement weather might bring about your demise, there is a better chance that you will live through the winter and go on to reproduce yourself. It is possible that seasonal depression may have been a valuable survival trait. Though it no longer serves any useful purpose, we are unfortunately stuck with it.

If you have seasonal depression, bright light therapy may help to reset your biological clock. Light therapy can be used alone but it is often used in conjunction with medications. Before you spend a lot of money on a phototherapy light or invest time sitting in front of one, you should obtain specific instructions that will increase the likelihood that the lights will be beneficial. The distance you sit from the light source, the intensity of the light, the amount of time you spend looking at it, and the time of day can all make a difference in the effectiveness of phototherapy. If you have a "reverse" seasonal pattern, feeling worse as the days grow *longer*, phototherapy lights will not be useful.

Electroconvulsive Therapy (ECT)

Psychotherapy can be helpful and will be discussed in a later section. Electroconvulsive therapy (ECT) is also a very effective treatment and can be useful in the unlikely situation that medications are not effective or well tolerated. ECT should also be considered if the depression is extremely severe or life threatening and a rapid response is needed. No one is certain exactly why ECT works, but it is known to affect the balance of numerous brain chemicals. It actually has a higher response rate and typically works faster than other available treatments for depression.

With all the medication choices that are now available, ECT is generally not considered first-line treatment, but it can be quite effective for a number of people. As with most forms of therapy, there can be some side effects including memory loss, but the loss of memory generally relates to events that take place right around the time of the treatments. There are many misconceptions about ECT, often perpetuated by misrepresentations in movies or television. It is helpful to turn to a professional for a more balanced discussion of ECT. It is not for everyone, but for some people, ECT can make all the difference in the world.

Transcranial Magnetic Stimulation is a technology that is being explored as a potential treatment option, but it is still investigational and is not available for general use.

Are "natural" treatments safe and effective?

Many people self-medicate with "natural" or herbal preparations that claim to be useful for a wide array of symptoms, such as depressed mood, fatigue, insomnia, and memory loss. Contrary to common beliefs, the "natural" origin of a product does not ensure its safety. These substances are not uniformly harmless.

Safety of these preparations is a big concern because the manufacturers are not required to determine side effects and potential toxicity prior to putting them on the market. The FDA does not have regulatory control over these substances unless it can be proven they are *not* safe. The manufacturers can claim that these preparations are beneficial for the health of certain organ systems or to treat many types of symptoms. They do not have to prove their claims. As long as the distributors do not claim that these preparations treat a specific *disease*, they can be classified as "dietary supplements" or "food additives" and are excluded from requirements to prove safety or effectiveness. Yet, when you consider the proposed uses for these preparations and the manner in which they are marketed, it becomes apparent that they only escape scrutiny as medications on a technicality. Even when the FDA suspects that a dietary supplement is harmful, its hands are tied until it can gather enough data to build a case against the substance. In the meanwhile, years may pass, people suffer from serious side effects or die, and in the end taxpayers, rather than manufacturers, foot the bill for the legal costs and research to prove that a substance is harmful.

Anything, even water—unquestionably a natural substance—has the potential to cause problems if excessive amounts are consumed at one time. A number of "natural" substances have been known to cause problems such as seizures, elevated heart rate or abnormal heart rhythm, high blood pressure, bleeding problems, confusion, agitation, liver failure, excessive sedation, hallucinations, and skin problems. For example, kava-kava has been associated with some cases of liver failure, and St. John's Wort can interfere with the effectiveness of medication used to prevent organ transplant rejection. Some preparations, when analyzed, have been found to be contaminated with over-the-counter and prescription drugs and dangerous substances such as lead and arsenic. Some herbal preparations do not contain the dosage that is printed on the bottle, and some contain none of the substance they claim to be providing.

The sale of herbal preparations is BIG business and it has been a very uncontrolled industry. There have probably been more studies on the safety of your toothpaste than on the safety of most of these treatments. Using anything that claims to be safe but has not been required to prove it is a bit like walking through the forest eating mushrooms without a good guidebook. Some of the choices may be just fine, but some may be big trouble. Keep in mind, if it sounds too good to be true, it usually is.

There are sometimes claims that "studies" have shown a preparation to be effective. The "scientific" data may even sound good because of the way scientific words, misleading information, and partial truths are woven into the presentation. In reality, there may not be any solid, reproducible evidence. Manufacturers don't bother with legitimate research because they are not required to do so, and it is very expensive. Just as you would question whether some highly advertised new-and-improved household product is really that great, it makes sense to question something you are about to put in your body, whether it is a standard medication or an herbal preparation. A healthy dose of skepticism allows you to be a more informed consumer. Although some preparations may be beneficial and safe, others may be ineffective or dangerous, and there is no sure way to know which description applies to any given herbal preparation. The medical community has begun to study some of these preparations, but it takes time to conduct good research. Even when a study has been done in a scientifically rigorous fashion, the evidence is not taken as gospel until other independent studies are able to replicate the findings.

Are herbal preparations chemically active?

"Natural" substances can certainly be pharmaco-logically active, and some of them may have potential benefits, but we don't have all of the information we need. There are a number of standard medications, which are clearly chemically active, that can be derived from natural sources. For example, digoxin (a heart medicine) can be derived from the Digitalis lanata (foxglove) plant. Digoxin can be lifesaving for a person in congestive heart failure, yet it can kill a person if the dose is too high. Aspirin-like substances can be derived from willow bark. Aspirin is a very useful medication to treat pain, prevent blood clotting, and decrease inflammation, but it's potentially dangerous for a person with a bleeding problem or an ulcer. This is the type of information we don't have for "natural" or "herbal" products. We don't know if they really do what they claim to do, we don't know about appropriate dosages, and we don't have a clear picture of associated risks, such as side effects, problems with other medical conditions, or interactions with other herbal substances or medications.

There are potential dangers in treating yourself

When people self-administer these preparations, there is no organized medical supervision or oversight to ascertain whether or not problems exist. A person without medical training might not have the experience and knowledge needed to identify a potentially serious side effect or medical problem. Even standard medications that have been through rigorous studies can produce a side effect that was not previously recognized, especially if it is a rare side effect. If enough doctors see an association between a drug and an unusual or adverse reaction, rare events can be identified. This doesn't happen when people are not under the supervision of a physician.

One final note about self-medicating with herbal preparations: If you have symptoms that are worrisome to you or are causing you a lot of problems, it makes sense to consult a physician rather than try to handle it on your own. Even doctors shouldn't self-medicate, because it is difficult to be objective and look at the big picture when you are trying to treat yourself. Self-diagnosis and treatment can cause problems and be a roadblock to getting appropriate and needed treatment.

3
Psychotherapy

Introduction

For some people the word "psychotherapy" conjures up an image of lying on a couch with a gentleman seated nearby stroking his beard and uttering statements such as "hmm . . . yes . . . tell me more. . . ." Movies and television have at times portrayed therapists and psychiatrists outlandishly, from the ultimately evil and/or corrupt to the outrageously seductive, from incredible buffoons to aloof or self-absorbed narcissists. Reality is, of course, much different from the movies. A television show about what most lawyers, police officers, or doctors really do, day in and day out, would not make for very enticing viewing. Likewise, an accurate portrayal of psychotherapy or therapists would not catch the attention of many viewers. Contrary to some movie portrayals, therapists are not all-knowing or all-powerful. They do not read your mind or interpret your every thought or action as something twisted and dysfunctional. Therapists are simply people who have training and expertise in helping others who are experiencing various emotional difficulties. Therapists do not necessarily focus solely on events from your childhood or try to uncover unconscious conflicts, although this may have been a more common approach in the past. Much of the psychotherapy that is done today is very focused on the here and now. A goal of therapy is to help you live well in the present. For some people, that *may* mean looking hard at the past but for virtually everyone in therapy it means looking for changes that can be made in the present. Therapy is about learning and change, among other things. Therapy can help you identify problems, habits, or patterns of thinking that may have contributed to or resulted from your depression.

Supportive Therapy

Early on in treatment people often benefit from some brief therapy that is primarily supportive in nature. Until the medications become effective, a person with depression may be lacking in the necessary energy and ability to process the information needed to participate in, and derive benefit from, other types of therapy. A therapist may be able to provide some coping tools, reassurance, advice, and a much-needed infusion of hope. The element of hope may be one of the most important components of therapy. Involvement of family members can be very helpful and education about depression is always beneficial.

Cognitive Therapy

At times, some people have viewed the mind, the brain and the body as separate entities, but they are very much interconnected. All of our observations of the world, all thoughts and feelings we experience, are translated into complex chemical reactions in our brains. Our experiences in the world and the way in which we conceptualize our experiences impact our brain chemistry. Likewise, brain chemistry affects our thoughts, emotions, behavior, and bodily functions. It goes both ways.

Cognitive therapy helps you to look at your thoughts and how they affect your feelings and behavior. Your thoughts may not be the cause of your depression, but they certainly can feed into the process and make you feel worse. If negative thoughts pop up in your brain and you automatically jump to the worst possible conclusions, interpreting events in a negative manner and misinterpreting the words and actions of other people, of course you are going to feel bad. For example, if your boss seems to give you a funny look at work, you might worry about your job performance then convince yourself that you are about to be fired. You may think through all the potential ramifications and before you know it, you become convinced that you are going to lose everything and find yourself homeless. You may construct a complete fantasy in your mind, and unless you dispel these thoughts, you will likely feel depressed and anxious. Your subsequent reactions to your boss may be influenced by these thoughts, compounding your problems. All of this can happen with the misinterpretation of just one look. You may never consider the possibility that your boss may have simply been suffering from indigestion or something else that has nothing to do with you.

Cognitive therapy is not just a matter of "thinking happy thoughts." Trying to "think happy thoughts" will not make you feel less depressed, but stepping back and looking at things more objectively and realistically can help. Cognitive therapy is not about pretending that everything is nice and rosy, but is more like taking off dark glasses and putting on clear lenses.

Behavioral Therapy

Behavioral therapy can address behavior patterns that feed into the depressive process, such as social withdrawal, isolation, and avoidance. This type of therapy may be helpful early on in treatment, even before a person is able to think clearly enough to benefit from cognitive therapy. "Cognitive behavioral therapy" is simply a combination of both cognitive techniques and behavioral strategies.

Interpersonal Therapy

Interpersonal therapy focuses on communication issues and current problems in relationships that may contribute to depression. Whether you have just developed depression or have had it for years, it influences your relationships with other people. Therapy can help you develop more productive strategies and skills and change unproductive or destructive behaviors.

Insight-oriented Therapy

Although many therapeutic approaches for depression involve short-term focused work on the present, some people may benefit from longer-term therapy. People sometimes have persistent destructive or self-defeating thought or behavior patterns that interfere with their lives. Identifying and addressing these patterns can lead to more satisfying experiences in the future.

While depression does not necessarily stem from past conflicts or trauma, sometimes people have had experiences that contribute to and perpetuate their depression. Unresolved problems from the past can interfere with future relationships, choices, decision-making, ability to cope with stressful life events, self-esteem, and ultimately a person's mood. You can't change the past, but you can work on changing the way the past affects you. Therapy can help you identify and work through painful issues, enabling you to come to some resolution, make changes if necessary and put things in perspective with regard to the person you are now.

Group Therapy

Many types of therapies can be presented in a group format. While the focus of various groups may differ, a common unifying thread is the validation and support that occurs in a group setting. Groups help provide people with concrete reassurance that they are not so different after all, and that other people are also struggling, even if from the outside they appear to be doing just fine. When groups of people are dealing with similar (but not necessarily identical) issues, there is the opportunity to learn from the experiences of the other people and gain a greater understanding of yourself and others. Groups help diminish social discomfort and isolation, and provide an opportunity to practice communication skills and work on relationships in a safe setting. Many people are initially nervous about being in group therapy, but keep in mind that the other people are in the same position. People who were initially reluctant to consider a group often later report that it was one of the best things they did for themselves.

"Eclectic" Therapy Strategies

Therapists often utilize their own individual blend of psychotherapeutic approaches that they have found useful. This is sometimes termed an "eclectic" approach, though there isn't anything that is known as "eclectic" therapy. This term basically means that a therapist may draw from different theoretical approaches and styles depending upon your particular circumstances and their areas of expertise.

What You Can Do for Yourself during a Depressive Episode

Try to keep a regular routine

Depression can cause a lot of disarray in people's lives, and an irregular schedule perpetuates the sense of chaos that many people experience. Try to maintain as regular a schedule as possible, including meals and sleep schedule, to help get your brain and body on the right track. Your routine doesn't have to be precisely the same every day, but try to avoid excess irregularity.

Try to have a balanced diet

Nutritional problems are rarely the causative factor for depressive symptoms, but when someone is depressed they often don't have a balanced diet. Some people have an increased intake of carbohydrates and sweets. Other people may not be hungry and simply forget to eat. People might need to force themselves to eat because the thought of food makes them feel ill. Preparing food or shopping for groceries may seem like a huge chore, so people often eat a lot of easy foods such as breakfast cereal. People will often grab a candy bar, cookie, or potato chips rather than sit down for a meal.

While there is no evidence that eating any particular kinds of foods will speed your recovery from depression, it is common sense that you will be healthier and feel better if you eat a reasonably balanced diet. When you are depressed, it can be easier to accomplish that goal if you keep it simple. You can buy prepared deli food (look for healthy selections), good quality frozen food, and ready-made sauces to accompany pasta. Try to avoid foods with excessive sugar, simple carbohydrates, and fat. Bring home a selection of easy-to-eat fruits and vegetables for snacking. People often buy fruits, but when they get home simply leave them in the bag, buried in the back of the refrigerator. If you wash the fruit right away and put it in a bowl on the table, you might be more likely to grab an apple, instead of reaching for the potato chips. If you feel so ill that you don't think you can force any food down, consider buying some nutritional shakes. It is often easier to drink than to eat. These shakes can be found in most large grocery stores and pharmacies. Once your stomach has settled down, you should try to eat regular well-balanced meals and snacks.

Although some people lose their appetite during a depressive episode, it is not unusual for people to experience an increase in appetite. If you eat as a way of trying to feel better or to comfort yourself, it may be helpful to see a therapist who can help you identify your emotional triggers for eating and work on healthier coping strategies. People often consume excessive sugar and calories by drinking soda pop or fruit juice. Switching to plain water can make a big difference in how you feel. A consultation with a nutritionist may help you work on making better food choices, without entirely giving up all the foods you love.

People often believe that vitamin supplementation can make up for poor nutrition, but vitamins are not a substitute for a well-balanced diet. If you are concerned about vitamin deficiency (and serious deficiencies are not very common in the U.S.), it is best to see a doctor to obtain recommendations about what might be healthy for you, rather than trying to manage it yourself. Many vitamins are safe to use, but taking excessive doses of certain vitamins, especially fat-soluble vitamins such as A, D, E, and K, can be risky because they become toxic at high levels. Water-soluble vitamins are less problematic, because they are more easily flushed out of your system. Minerals can also be a problem for some people. While iron may be beneficial to women who lose a lot of blood during menstruation, people with a family history of hemachromatosis (a disease in which cells get overloaded with iron) may need to be very careful to avoid excessive iron. Again, an excessive amount of anything is seldom beneficial and can, in some cases, be dangerous.

Try to develop healthy sleep habits

Many people struggle with insomnia during a depressive episode. If you are having trouble falling asleep at night, try to do something relaxing before bedtime. You should avoid doing work or getting into intense discussions right before bedtime, as these can interfere with relaxation. Exercising several hours before bedtime can improve your sleep, whereas exercise right before bedtime is stimulating. Having a hot bath a couple of hours before bedtime, then allowing your body to cool down, can help promote sleep. Smoking, drinking alcohol, and consuming caffeine are detrimental to your sleep. Don't go to bed hungry but don't eat excessively before bedtime either. Avoid using your bed for activities other than sleep and sexual activity, such as watching television or doing paperwork. If you aren't feeling sleepy, you may want to try relaxing a bit longer before lying down, otherwise you might end up just laying in bed, wide awake, worrying about whether you are going to fall asleep or not. As much as possible, try to go to bed and wake up at about the same time each day, even on weekends; a routine helps regulate your body rhythms.

One of the most common sleep problems during depression is waking up in the middle of the night, once or many times, sometimes at nearly the exact same time. If you can't get back to sleep within fifteen to twenty minutes, get up and do something relaxing for a while, such as reading or listening to calming music, then go to bed again as soon as you start to feel sleepy. You don't want to lie in bed, watching the clock, wondering if you are going to be able to fall asleep and worrying about how little time there is left to sleep. Lying there for hours at a time, night after night, may train your brain to think that beds are for "not" sleeping, and in the future it may become even more difficult to fall asleep in your bed. It is better to get up and do some quiet activity, being careful not to get too involved in what you are doing, since your main objective is to get back to sleep.

Conversely, some people with depression crave sleep and could practically sleep around the clock. Rather than waking up feeling refreshed, however, people generally wake up feeling just as exhausted as when they went to bed. The extra sleep does not contribute to a sense of well-being and it can make it next to impossible to get anything done. Depression also tends to worsen if too much time is spent lying alone in a dark room with your head under the covers.

Many people with depression lie down at night, only to have thoughts swirl around in their heads, making it impossible to fall asleep. If this happens to you, remind yourself that you can think about these things in the morning, or keep a notebook by your bedside so that you can quickly jot down a brief note. You can't resolve anything in the middle of the night. If you can clear the thoughts out of your head, you will have a better chance of falling asleep. If you find that worrisome thoughts frequently pop up at bedtime, you may want to set aside a specific "worry time" during the daytime hours. Then at night, you can remind yourself that you will think about those things at the specified hour. Once your depression is treated, you probably won't be plagued by this problem anymore.

It's not possible to control exactly when you fall asleep, but you do have some control over when you wake up (even though it may seem impossible to drag yourself out of bed). People often feel like they have just fallen into a good sleep when it is time to get up. It can be difficult, but waking up at the same time every day, even if you have not slept well the previous night, will help keep your sleep/wake cycles more stable. Even if you are very tired during the day, it is generally advisable to minimize napping. Naps may throw off your schedule and interfere with your body's drive to sleep at night. If you feel like you must take a nap, set an alarm for one hour so that you don't sleep for an extended period.

It is not unusual for people to stay up very late, spending time on the Internet, watching television, or just putzing around. This may help people to distract themselves from negative thoughts or feelings. It may be the only chance for people to finally have time to themselves. While some people are exhausted early in the evening, others find that nighttime is when they finally feel awake, have some energy, and can think clearly. Staying up late, however, feeds into social isolation and causes sleep deprivation. Irritability, fatigue, and poor concentration can result from this behavior. Unfortunately, it is difficult to set limits on these activities. People get carried away and before they know it, the hour is quite late. Then, even if they are able to fall asleep, there are simply not enough hours remaining before they have to get up. The next day is worse because they are even more sleep deprived; yet, the same thing happens night after night. Getting a good night's sleep does not cure depression, but having a bad night of sleep can make you feel a lot worse.

Most people need some quiet time for themselves, but if you are staying up late to try to have some "alone" time, your well-being may suffer. It may seem next to impossible, but it is worth trying to carve out time during the day, rather than depriving yourself of sleep.

Avoid alcohol and drugs

Alcohol and drugs do not mix well with depression. These substances can act as depressants and perpetuate the illness, as well as interfere with treatment. Alcohol and drugs, even in amounts that you would not normally think of as causing a problem, can be problematic if you have depression. Acute alcohol intoxication can be dangerous because it is more likely for a distraught person to act impulsively on suicidal thoughts.

People sometimes use alcohol to help them fall asleep. What many people do not know is that even if alcohol causes grogginess initially, it disturbs sleep in the middle of the night. You do not get good quality sleep after consuming alcohol. This can happen with just one beer, one glass of wine or one mixed drink before bedtime.

Alcohol is sometimes used to make a person feel more at ease and comfortable around others, but it doesn't help people to develop social skills, and more often leads to behavior that is regretted.

Many people use drugs and alcohol as forms of "self-medication": to boost their mood, decrease tension and anxiety, and feel more "normal." Alcohol or drugs might seem to help "take the edge off" temporarily, but the net effect is increased depression. People who experience a sense of relief after using alcohol or some other substance may fall into the trap of escalating alcohol or drug use. A person often feels worse the day after using a substance, and in order to feel better, at least temporarily, they use it again.

People don't start using alcohol or drugs with the objective of developing a problem, but that is exactly what can happen. After a while, it can be difficult to ascertain which came first, depression or an alcohol problem. People try to hide their problem and end up carrying around a lot of shame. Many people find themselves in this situation, and it doesn't mean they are bad or weak. If you think that you have developed a problem, it can be a relief to talk with someone about it. It can also be a new beginning.

In the past, depression was generally not treated until a person abstained from alcohol for four to six weeks, with the rationale that it could take that long for the depressive effects of alcohol to be reversed. Waiting to start antidepressants could help differentiate primary depression from the depression caused by the effects of alcohol on the brain. Unfortunately, it is often difficult for a person who has an underlying depression and alcoholism to attain sobriety unless both problems are treated simultaneously. If significant depression is present when a person enters alcohol treatment, antidepressants are now often prescribed concurrently, at the beginning of alcohol cessation. Later it can be determined if there is the need for ongoing treatment with medication.

Try to exercise

Exercise may not cure depression, but it does help many people feel better. Even if you are a person who does not get an immediate boost from exercise, it can decrease feelings of irritability and help you feel physically better in the long run. It is often hard to get started, but it's easier if you begin with reasonable expectations. Try to talk yourself into walking for just a couple of minutes. Later you can talk yourself into walking an extra block or two. Work up gradually to improve your chances of sticking with it. If you set your goals too high initially, you are less likely to get started or to sustain that pace. Exercise equipment and health club memberships may be great, but if you can't bring yourself to use them, they won't help. You might be less likely to postpone exercising if you find someone to accompany you regularly. Try to identify some form of exercise you might actually enjoy, rather than picking an activity that bores you to tears. If getting started with an exercise program has been an obstacle, try walking. It is a natural daily activity for most people and it is a beginning.

Try to overcome inertia

People often become less involved in activities during depression, and the inactivity, boredom, and decreased productivity can make everything seem worse. You may think it's pointless to try to do anything because you can't conceive of anything being enjoyable or helping you feel better. It can be extremely hard to get anything done; even getting out of bed can be a chore. You may feel immobilized, but this does not mean that you are lazy. The part of your brain responsible for initiating activity may not be functioning well; the spark that gets you started is missing. You may feel like you have to overcome an energy barrier in order to get started on a task. Like pushing a car, it's hard work at first and it may seem like you're not making much progress, but once you get it moving, the momentum builds. Ultimately, doing things can help you feel better.

Accomplish tasks by setting reasonable goals

When everything seems like an effort, procrastination can become habitual. The procrastination causes disorganization and guilt, which feed into the depressive process. One way to overcome inertia is to break down tasks into smaller more manageable units. Try doing part of a task or working for a set amount of time rather than trying to do it all at once. Accomplishments, no matter how small, can help you feel better.

Limit the quantity of work that you set out to do

If you have to wash laundry, talk yourself into putting in one load rather than thinking you have to do it all. If you have to fold laundry, set a goal of folding a few pieces rather than the whole basket. If you have a stack of mail to open, just open one or two envelopes, and don't bother to open the obvious junk mail. Just throw it out. Many people avoid paying bills because it seems too hard, even if they have enough money in the bank. If you have bills that are stacking up simply because you feel unable to deal with them, open just one envelope and take care of it. Write out one check, or start by writing the due date on the outside of the envelope. These are just some examples, but try to apply this principle to whatever it is that you need or want to accomplish. For almost everything, one step at a time usually works best.

Limit the amount of time you spend on a task

It's much easier to talk yourself into doing something if you put a limit on the amount of time you are going to spend on the task. If you aim to complete everything at once, you may become overwhelmed and not start anything. Once started, you may lose track of time or find yourself distracted. If you instead plan to spend a few minutes on a task, maybe even set a timer, you will make a dent in it and eventually accomplish more than if you had tried to do it all at once.

Give yourself credit for your accomplishments

Once you have done what you set out to do, try not to discount your efforts by telling yourself that you should have been able to do better. Remember, you wouldn't expect someone who is recovering from a heart attack to get right back up and start a marathon. If you had a serious spinal cord injury, being able to wiggle your toes would be cause for celebration. Depression can immobilize people too. Your small victories are a triumph when you consider what you are up against. You may need some time to get back in the swing of things, but eventually it is going to happen. Don't beat yourself up for what you haven't been able to do yet. You need to recognize your small successes and tell yourself "good job."

Plan your day

People often feel at loose ends during a depression, and don't know what to do with themselves or how to fill their time. Adding some structure to your day can help you feel more in control. Set one small goal for the morning, afternoon, and evening. Remember, these should be limited goals so that you have a good chance of actually accomplishing them. The morning tasks may be getting up, showering, brushing your teeth, getting dressed, and eating something. The afternoon activity could be taking a five-minute walk. In the evening you could do a time-limited task around the house. Start small and gradually work your way up.

Allow yourself the opportunity to do things for enjoyment—make time for play and relaxation

There might not be much that sounds enjoyable or interesting right now, but try to think of things that once brought you pleasure. This can be an important way to reconnect with your world. Once you force yourself to do something, you may feel a bit better, even if you weren't looking forward to the activity. You might be surprised by a brief feeling of satisfaction or pleasure. Even if you don't feel any pleasure, the distraction of doing something can help take your mind off the way you feel. Every little bit helps. Taking time to relax and doing pleasurable activities is healthy for you and necessary for a balanced life.

Chip away at social isolation

People with depression often do not want to be around other people; there is a tendency to withdraw and isolate oneself. Most people need some human interaction, and though you don't have to be a social butterfly, making connections with other people can help you feel less depressed. The more you stay secluded in your home, the more anxious you will feel about leaving.

It is not unusual to feel nervous, insecure, or at a loss for words around other people. It's okay if you are not the life of the party. Just being around other people can be good for you, even if you don't have much to say. Once you get out among other people, you may find that you are less uncomfortable than you thought you would be.

If you are worried about what to say to people if they ask how you've been doing, prepare a few stock phrases ahead of time, such as "I've been through a rough spell, but I'm hanging in there," or "I've had some health problems, but things are improving." If you are exchanging social pleasantries with someone you hardly know it may be appropriate to avoid being put on the spot by simply saying "I'm okay. How have you been doing?" If you worry that people will probe for details, remember that you can always say something like "Thanks for asking. I appreciate your concern, but I really don't care to talk about it."

Being irritable and becoming easily annoyed is common in depression, and feeling this way can make it difficult for you to be around other people. Large numbers of people or excessive noise can be over-stimulating and overwhelming. If you are concerned about demanding social situations, you might want to choose activities that are more low-key. Rather than going to a large social event where you'll be expected to make a lot of small talk, try something less stressful like going out for coffee or going to a movie. Take a walk with someone. Many people don't want to commit to doing anything because they are afraid they'll feel awful and won't be able to escape. Sometimes it's easier to think about doing something if you plan an "out" for yourself. Give yourself permission to leave early if you've had enough. You can let people know ahead of time that you may only be able to stay for a little while. When you manage to go somewhere, it's often a better experience than you had imagined it would be. Engaging with other people allows you the opportunity for some rewarding experiences, whereas there is zero potential if you are at home, in bed.

Pick up the phone and make one telephone call. Say yes to one social activity, even if you aren't thrilled about participating. It will likely be better than you anticipate.

Habits

Many people busy themselves with activities that require little thought, such as television, computer or video games, the internet, shopping, eating, gambling, or endless housework in order to escape or feel more in control. In moderation, these pasttimes may not be a problem, but when they are pursued to the exclusion of other more fulfilling or important activities, they can cause problems in your life and serve to further isolate you. People may while away the hours with some of these activities, staying up far too late. If you have found that you are overly preoccupied with these sorts of habits, it may be helpful to put limits on them. If you are "stuck in a rut," a therapist can help you work on strategies for changing nonproductive or self-destructive habits.

Stay in the present

Depression has a way of robbing people of their ability to live in the present. You are powerless to change the past or control the future, and it's easy to get despondent and overwhelmed if you are inundated with thoughts about events beyond the "here and now."

Don't look too far ahead

As much as possible, try not to spend too much time thinking or worrying about the future. Keep in mind that there may not be much you can do about it right now. Try to focus on today, the next hour, or even the next minute. You can't take care of everything at once, but you can take things one step at a time. Concentrate on doing something about some of the current stresses in your life. Focusing on the present, while it is happening, will help you feel more in control and better prepared to deal with events that come your way in the future.

Avoid getting stuck in the past

A frequent component of depression is becoming pre-occupied with the past. Depression casts past events in a negative light and causes self-doubt. You may recall bad things that happened and painful memories more readily. You may review mistakes that you have made or feel troubled by things you have said or done, even if you weren't concerned at the time. Events that other people didn't give a second thought to, long-forgotten incidents, may come back to haunt you. Negative thoughts can go round and around in your mind without you getting anywhere with them. Past events you thought you had come to terms with may seem brand new in your mind again. Old wounds may open up and seem as intensely painful as when they first happened. If you can keep your feet firmly planted in the present and work on the here and now, you will feel more in control.

While there isn't any way to change the past, you can work on changing the way you think about it and the way it affects you. Cognitive behavioral therapy, which is discussed in the section on psychotherapy, can help you look at your thoughts more rationally. Once your depression lifts, you may find that some of the issues that you thought were critical have faded away because they were a product of the depression. The opposite is also true. Once you are better, you may realize that there are other problems that you didn't know existed, because your depression clouded everything. Depression can mask problems, and when the depression lifts, you can more clearly identify areas in your life that really could use some work. You are able to make healthier choices and positive changes in your life.

Avoid negative experiences

Now is not the time to delve into deep, dark, disturbing books or movies. Focus on more lighthearted material, even if you don't feel lighthearted. If everything you hear on the news or read in the newspapers is gloomy, set them aside; it's hard enough to deal with those things when you are feeling good. It's time to take a break from negative experiences in general, at least for a while. If certain people in your life tend to be overly critical or sarcastic, you may need to minimize contact with them for now, though you should be careful not to make rash decisions about relationships.

Place emphasis on things that go right (rather than things that go wrong)

If you catalog everything in your life that seems to have gone wrong, you will feel worse. During depression there is a tendency to focus on the negative side of things more than you would under normal circumstances. Instead of keeping tabs on the things that go wrong or the times you feel bad, try to take note of small things that went right or brought you a moment of pleasure. Jot down anything that was the least bit enjoyable or gave you a feeling of accomplishment, anything that made you feel even a little bit good, even if only for a short time.

Try not to make major decisions

People often think that if they changed something externally in their lives, such as their job, relationships, or home, their depression would go away. Since depression can influence the way you think and perceive, it is often prudent to postpone major decisions until you feel better. You might have considered quitting your job, leaving your relationship, or moving, but once the depression has lifted you might see things differently. Those decisions can always be made later. If drastic changes or decisions are made in the middle of depression, you might burn bridges and later have regrets. Trying to literally move away from your problems (also referred to as a "geographical cure") can mean that you find yourself in an unfamiliar environment. The stress of being in a new environment can make it even more difficult to cope, and you simply take your problems with you. Quitting a job or leaving a relationship can be equally devastating. In some situations, changes may be helpful, but most of the time it is advisable to delay these decisions until you are feeling stable and able to think more clearly.

Don't drive if you are distracted

If your concentration is impaired and you don't feel safe driving, you aren't safe. It isn't always easy to stay focused on the road, monitor traffic and remember all the details involved in driving if depression has affected your concentration and memory. Better to have someone else drive you, no matter how inconvenient it is, rather than to risk injury or death for yourself and others. Once your depression is better you should be able to focus and drive safely again.

Ways to Decrease Your Susceptibility to Depression

Certain thought patterns and behaviors can increase stress

Certain thought patterns and behaviors can make a person more vulnerable to getting "stressed out" and prone to becoming depressed. These are often long-standing patterns but may become even more pronounced during a depressive episode. It's not necessary, or even possible, to fix all of these problems right away. As you start to feel better, though, it can be helpful to identify and modify things that might contribute to your depression. Talking with a therapist is often the most effective way to help you make progress in these areas.

Try to worry less about what other people think

Being overly critical of yourself, trying to constantly please others, constantly seeking reassurance, or letting your self-esteem be dependent upon other people's opinions can set you up to feel bad. Depression can make you tend to worry more about what other people think of you. Other people are typically unaware that you place so much emphasis on their opinion. You may misinterpret what others say and do, thinking that they have a low opinion of you. You may judge yourself harshly and believe that other people do as well. Depression can leave you feeling inadequate, thinking that you are worthless and different from other people. Depression distorts your view of yourself. If you fear criticism, you may overcompensate and try to win approval by doing more for people, then end up feeling resentful, unappreciated, and overwhelmed. You may allow others to unjustly criticize you because you don't feel good about yourself.

It is okay to say NO

If you have a hard time saying NO to people, it's likely that you will find yourself overcommitted and in over your head. You may put pressure on yourself to do too much, so much that you can't possibly handle everything on your plate, and then pay a high personal toll. If you have taken on more than you can realistically accomplish, you will probably end up feeling unhappy. Your reserves may be empty. You can't do it all, so you avoid it. When you don't follow through with fulfilling your obligations, you end up feeling guilty and depressed. It is better to apply yourself more fully to a few activities than to spread yourself so thin that you can't feel successful at anything.

Bear in mind that even if people ask you to do something for them, it doesn't necessarily mean that you have to do it, that they expect you to do it, or that they will think less of you if you don't. If you have always been known for saying yes, saying no might surprise people because they have been trained to expect a yes. Sometimes you have to say "No thank-you" to people who mean well but who may not have an accurate idea about what is best for you. If a person can't accept this or if their opinion of you depends upon what you do for them, it is probably best to firmly say no. You don't need that kind of relationship with anyone. You can't please everyone and that is okay.

Before you say YES, think about whether you want to do what has been asked of you and whether or not you have the energy to do it. If you are doing something just because you think you should or to please someone else, you may want to reconsider. If you are known for self-sacrifice or being overly responsible, learning to say no can be a healthy new habit. Taking care of yourself and placing importance on your own needs is not selfish. You don't have to give endlessly of yourself in order to be a worthwhile, caring, and giving person. Each of us has our own limits, and learning where to draw the line can be more productive, and healthy. If it is hard to say NO in the moment, it is okay to stall until you've had a chance to think about it. Try to think of some stock answers that you can use when you are put on the spot, such as "I'll get back to you" or "I need to think about it" or "I need to check my calendar" or "I have to see if I have a previous commitment." If you know it is something that you do not want to do, you can give a "thanks for thinking of me, but I really can't" type of answer.

Anger and conflict resolution

Anger is a normal human emotion. It occurs for many reasons, but is often caused by a failure of communication, distortion or misinterpretation of another person's words or actions, or two people having different expectations in a given situation. Many people do not recognize their feelings of anger. People are often afraid of anger or don't know what to do with it. There may be fear of losing control or worry about the reaction of the other person. Instead of always letting anger lead to negative experiences, such as heated arguments, it can be helpful to learn to recognize that you are angry before you react. If you can first identify the reason for your anger, it is possible to work on ways to deal with it appropriately. You can turn it into something healthier: an opportunity to work on resolving a problem. Anger and irritability are often accentuated by depression, and treating the depression can make a world of difference.

Avoiding conflict and "stuffing" anger can be a problem

Frankly, many people prefer to avoid dealing with conflict. Anger is an uncomfortable emotion. However, if you manage conflict and anger by avoidance, you shut down the possibility of coming to any resolution. Perhaps you react by not talking at all. You may harbor grudges and resentments, which can eat away at you, or perhaps you funnel your anger into sarcastic or critical comments. You may react disproportionately to something that is trivial. If your anger resurfaces later, out of context and disconnected from the original event, your behavior will be viewed as inappropriate to the situation. All of these behaviors can erode your relationships and be destructive to your emotional well-being.

Talking about problems doesn't always have to lead to lengthy discussions or arguments; it may be sufficient to briefly tell a person how you feel in a particular situation and let them know your thoughts. Other people can't really know what is on your mind unless you spell it out.

Assertiveness

Depression often causes people to be risk aversive. You may feel safer sticking with what is known to you, even if you know that the status quo is not healthy for you. You may be leery of speaking your mind, reticent in interpersonal relationships. You may worry about other people's reactions, seek approval or feel vulnerable to potential criticism. You may be uncertain of yourself. As a result, you may clam up and not say or do anything, even when you are feeling very frustrated or angry.

If you work on ways to express your thoughts in the present, as things happen, you are less likely to feel misunderstood and slighted. You may also gather valuable insights about the other person's perspective. Misunderstandings often occur because people make different (and sometimes erroneous) assumptions about a situation. If you think that it won't do any good to say anything, you may give up without trying. This is the start of a self-fulfilling prophecy. Other people will have no idea about what is on your mind and you won't resolve anything. Nothing will change if you don't speak up. Other people may not always respond in the way that you would like them to, but it is more likely that they will if you tell them what you are thinking. Give them a chance to meet you half way. If things don't work out the way you wanted, at least you can feel better knowing that you tried.

Try to discuss your anger when you have calmed down

Anger is best dealt with directly and, though it may seem to be a contradiction in terms, calmly. It doesn't help to stuff it but it also doesn't help if you go on a rampage. "Letting it all out," yelling and screaming, is not a healthy release; angry explosions make matters worse and are a barrier to effective communication and problem solving. Expressing anger in this way is often just an attempt to hurt the other person as much as possible. We have all felt this way at one time or another, but raging at someone prevents you from really dealing with the problem. It may feel good in the moment, but it isn't respectful, it doesn't help the situation, or promote understanding and change. The guilt you may experience later will not help you to feel good about yourself either.

Some ways to have a fair argument

1. Don't "ambush" the other person with your anger. If people are taken by surprise, they are more likely to react defensively, making it difficult to accomplish anything. Try to calmly let them know that you are feeling angry and what you are angry about.

2. Let yourself cool down before starting the discussion. If you aren't cooled down yet, pick a different agreed-upon time that is not too far into the future.

3. Limit the discussion to one incident that made you angry rather than getting side-tracked and venting all of your frustrations from the past. Don't use your anger about the current situation as an opportunity to clobber the other person with all the things that have ever made you angry. Decide what is the most important thing you want to discuss and what kinds of goals you have for the discussion.

4. Don't belittle the other person. Avoid loud angry tones, derogatory comments, sarcasm, and name-calling. This is disrespectful and will only lead to defensiveness and more anger.

5. Don't monopolize the conversation. Each person should allow the other person opportunities to talk, and they should be allowed to speak without interruption.

6. Try to listen to what the other person is saying. If you are preoccupied with what you are going to say next, while they are

talking, you won't really be able hear what is said. If you don't completely understand what someone is trying to say, ask the person to explain it again. Pay attention to the other person's physical and emotional responses.

7. Avoid telling the other person that they *always do this* or *never do that.* Overgeneralizations are rarely true and tend to shift the focus of the conversation, getting you off track into arguments about past issues. The other person may feel the need to invalidate the "always" or "never" statements and you may try to back up your statement with examples, none of which really pertains to the issue at hand. And since it is not unusual for one person to recall past events differently than another person, you could argue endlessly and never come to any resolution.

8. Rather than telling the other person that they make you feel a certain way, tell them that you feel a certain way (sad, hurt, angry) when they do what is bothering you. They don't have the power to create your feelings; feelings come from inside yourself. No one can make you feel or

behave in a certain way and likewise, you can't make someone else feel or behave in a certain way.

9. Try to avoid the words "should" or "shouldn't." Those words sound controlling and don't allow for an open discussion. Rather than telling someone what they should have done, tell them what you wish would or would not have happened.

10. Try to look at things from the other person's perspective. If you step back and think about how the other person might think or feel about a certain situation, it is easier to understand why they respond the way they do. This allows you to view the other person as a person, rather than as an opponent, and make positive changes in the way you interact. You do not necessarily need to agree with the other person, but acknowledging another person's point of view or simply saying that you didn't realize that something bothered them so much can completely change the character of a discussion.

11. Never try to have a serious discussion if either of you is tired, hungry, or intoxicated. You will not be able to think clearly

or focus on the discussion. You may say things that you don't really mean, making the situation worse.

12. If the discussion gets out of control, tempers flare, or it's just not productive, stop and agree to a time when you will pick up the discussion again. Leave rather than getting into a fighting match. Physical threats, intimidation, or violence is never okay. There is *no* justification for violent behavior. If someone says that you deserved physical punishment, they are wrong. If you feel unsafe or feel like you might be violent towards the other person, remove yourself from the situation immediately.

13. A good rule of thumb is "it's not whether you win or lose, it's how you play the game." Your relationship is not going to be healthy if one or both of you feels the need to "win" the argument. Having a winner and loser in competitive sports is part of the landscape, but in relationships it certainly does not promote healthy interaction. No one truly comes out ahead if the focus is winning. It is more productive to clarify the problem, try to understand the other person's point of view, and work

on problem solving. In the end, it is possible that you may simply end up agreeing
to disagree, and that can be okay. If you are
able to come to a mutual understanding,
it can be even better. Compromise on
both sides may be necessary and desirable.
Either way, your relationship is on more
solid ground if you can respect the other
person's point of view.

You don't have to be perfect (none of us are)

A tendency towards perfectionism can get the best of
you. It's hard enough if you have perfectionist tenden-
cies to begin with, but if you have depression, the drive
for perfection can be amplified. You may feel like you
are not worthwhile unless you do things perfectly or
are the "best." If being less than perfect means that you
have "failed," then you will not feel successful at much
of anything. No one is perfect and nothing is done "perfectly." Perfection is an elusive, impossible goal. There
are endless variations in the way in which something
can be done. Who can judge which is the best?

Perfectionism interferes with your ability to recognize things that you have done well. It can prevent
you from starting and finishing tasks. It holds you
back from being as productive or creative as you

might otherwise be. Thinking that you have to make "perfect" choices and fear of making a "wrong" decision can prevent you from making any decision. Part of growth and learning is to do something, and then consider what you might do differently next time. If you strive for perfection, there may not be a "next time" because you don't even allow yourself the opportunity to have a "this time." Your fear of failure can hold you back. If you can be satisfied with doing a "good enough" job, you will probably be much more relaxed and do better work in the long run. Small imperfections rarely ruin the whole experience, unless you let them. Even if you make a big mistake, you aren't alone. We all make mistakes, big and small. Try to learn from it and move on, rather than beating yourself up.

You may fear that if you are not perfect, other people will criticize you or show disapproval, but who among us can realistically expect perfection? What you do, whether it is your job, a project at home, or some other endeavor, does not determine how valuable you are as a person.

It may help to try to identify fears that underlie your perfectionism and bring them out in the open. You can then examine them rationally. Pose questions such as, "What is the worst thing that can happen if I don't do it perfectly?" "How likely is it that the worst will happen?" and "To what extent would I be hurt if the worst did happen?" If your perfectionism is made worse by depression, which is often the case, you will be less prone to these unrealistic expectations once your depression is treated.

Practice healthy detachment; let go of things you can't control

People often feel upset and stressed by thinking that they have a responsibility to fix things that are beyond their control, but there is so much we simply can't control. Worrying about things you cannot change can make you feel like a nervous wreck, under enormous pressure in impossible situations. The end result may be frustration, anger, depression, anxiety, fatigue, and helplessness. People are sometimes socialized to believe that they must "fix things" for others. Learning that this isn't true can be a liberating revelation.

Acknowledging that you have no real power to change another person's behavior can set you free. If something isn't under your control, you are helpless to fix the situation. You are not, however, helpless to alter your response. Figuring out what is or isn't your problem, then letting go of things you can't control, can ultimately help you feel less burdened. Doing so allows you the freedom to focus on things that you can influence, rather than wasting your time in a futile pursuit or feeling depressed about things you cannot change.

Feel your own feelings

If you have trouble determining the boundary between someone else's problems and your own, you can get caught in the trap of letting their misfortune or behavior influence your emotional state. If someone else is happy, you are happy. If someone is sad, so are you. If they are angry, you may feel responsible and want to make it right for them. The end result is a chaotic emotional life. By focusing your attention on other people, you also avoid looking at your own issues. This may feel more comfortable in the short term, but doing so prevents you from making changes that can help you in the long run.

Try to avoid guilt, shame, and blame

Shame and guilt don't do you or anyone else much good, but these feelings are very common, and often intensify, during a depressive episode. People often have a distorted view of themselves and magnify even their smallest shortcomings. You might "beat yourself up" about something you have said or done, feel excessively guilty, or replay painful memories over and over in your head. Negative thoughts pop unbidden into your mind. You might feel like every bad thing that happens is your fault. Once you have been treated for depression, these kinds of thoughts will likely diminish. In the meantime, while waiting for the depression to get better, you can concentrate on letting go of these thoughts as they occur.

Depression can make you susceptible to erroneous thoughts that you are a miserable and unworthy person, a failure as a human being who deserves to suffer. These types of thoughts can prevent you from doing anything to help yourself. If you feel stuck in these patterns, it can be helpful to see a therapist.

On the other hand, when people have depression there is sometimes a tendency to project blame onto other people. If you pick out small faults, become overly critical, and make mountains out of molehills, people may tiptoe around you and feel like they are walking on eggshells. You may send the message that you think another person is responsible for making you feel bad, but your bad mood isn't anyone's fault. If you feel crabby, you might convince yourself that it's because of the way someone else is acting. There is a natural tendency to look for an external reason for feeling bad. These thoughts cause a paralysis of action, however, because it's hard to do anything to make yourself feel better if you think your bad moods or problems are always because of someone else. You can begin to help yourself once you recognize that the only person you can truly do anything about is yourself.

If, realistically, someone or something else is

directly affecting your emotional state, it helps to recognize it and to figure out what you can do. You may not be able to change a situation or another person's behavior, but you can work on your response. Rather than viewing yourself as a victim of circumstances, work on recognizing that you have choices; this change in mindset can be empowering. If someone consistently treats you poorly, you can decide whether or not to continue the relationship. Some of the choices may be difficult, but you do have choices.

Work on letting go of little things

Life is full of stresses, big and small. Try not to fret about everyday annoyances and things that are not important in the grand scheme of things. This is difficult, because depression causes crankiness, and small irritants or stresses can seem magnified. There is a tendency to react with exaggerated and irrational responses. Ask yourself how important a given situation really is. Remind yourself that depression can amplify everything. Try to decide if it is worth your energy or whether you need to just move past it. Does it really matter to you? Is your level of anger or distress justifiable? How important will it be tomorrow, next week, or a year from now? Is it something that is going to eat at you and continue to bother you? If so, you should deal with it. Give yourself some time to think about it, and then if it is truly important, do something about it. If, on the other hand, it isn't very important, let it go rather than stew about it.

If you feel irritable, you might ease the tension by letting people know that you're feeling edgy, then give yourself a little time away to let things settle down. Practice distracting yourself in some way before you react. If you need to leave the room to cool down, do it. The more you are able to minimize impulsive, angry comments, the better.

Driving recklessly is an unhealthy emotional release

First and foremost, driving on public roads is a mode of transportation. The highways are for everyone to use. For some people, driving provides a release and an emotional thrill. Driving up fast behind another person and hugging their bumper to try to get them to move over can give people a sense of power. Some people are "addicted" to the feeling they get when they are driving fast, not unlike the feeling a gambler might have when playing for high stakes. Unfortunately, when played out on public highways, the stakes *are* high and include the risk of death for innocent bystanders. The death of a baby, small child, or *anyone* is not worth that rush of adrenaline you might get out of driving fast. Better to take up amateur racing, skydiving, bike racing, or some other legitimate sport rather than risk killing someone. Denial runs deep and people often believe that this will not happen when they are driving, but it can and it does. Emotional driving is always a mistake.

If you find yourself feeling exasperated and angry with other drivers, try taking a deep breath. Try to put yourself in their place. The other driver might be a teenager, driving on the freeway for the first time. Perhaps they are feeling ill, driving a pregnant woman to the hospital, or trying to deal with noise from a carload of children. Perhaps they just made a mistake; we all do at times. Whatever the case, that person is a human being, someone who other people care about. That person could be someone you care about. They aren't driving poorly just to make you miserable. If you respond to other peoples' mistakes by driving aggressively, you are endangering yourself and others. If you scream and curse or make threatening gestures, you are going to feel more agitated. The other driver may become frightened and panic. Accidents often happen when drivers let their emotions get the best of them, and no one deserves to die just because they made a mistake. If you really think about that other person as another human being, it's more difficult to justify your rage. Even if the other driver is obviously rude, careless, or overaggressive, you can't teach them common courtesy or proper driving skills by driving aggressively in return. If the other person is driving slower than you would like them to, have a talk with yourself. It won't be the end of the world if your car trip takes an additional minute or two because someone was a pokey driver. Take a deep breath and count slowly . . . and let it go. If you can manage your anger, you will feel more relaxed when you get where you are going. Most importantly, everyone will arrive safely.

Work on recognizing when you are feeling overwhelmed

When people have depression, they often become accustomed to pushing forward regardless of how lousy they feel. You may be good at putting on your "public face" in order to go about your daily life. Staying active is preferable to lying immobilized in bed, but if you're used to putting one foot in front of the other even when you feel bad, you may not recognize how bad things are until you feel like you have run into a brick wall and can't take it anymore. Being able to recognize the signs that things are not going well can help you prevent yourself from slipping down the slope to the bottom of the hill. Try to look back and figure out your personal warning signs, then try to manage the stressors before they get the best of you. Before you get to the breaking point, take some time out for yourself. When you're feeling stuck or stressed, take a break. Take a walk, exercise, listen to music, relax, meditate or read—whatever helps you just get away from it all for a while.

Avoid avoidance

Many people who have had depression for a long time fall into the trap of habitual procrastination—avoiding even simple tasks and obligations because everything feels difficult. Unfortunately, even when the depression lifts this tendency may remain. Avoidance can become ingrained behavior and the consequences of avoiding important activities are significant. People can feel stressed, overwhelmed, and guilt-ridden, which in turn can make a person more prone to getting depressed. Chapter four introduced some strategies for getting started on tasks and activities. However, if you are having trouble initiating changes or being consistent, it is often helpful to work with a therapist. Learning to tackle tasks promptly can leave you feeling less stressed and give you more time to do the things you truly want to do.

Time management

Life will feel more chaotic and you will feel more stressed if you chronically run behind schedule, are late for appointments, or have difficulty accomplishing tasks in the amount of time you have set aside. The first step in addressing this problem is to identify the factors that feed into this pattern.

If you have a tendency to try to accomplish "one more thing" before leaving for a scheduled appointment, there is a good chance that you will lose track of time and leave late, even if you had ample time to begin with. Retraining yourself will require planning and organization, but it is possible to change and the pay-off is well worth the time invested. Start by making a reasonable guess about how long it will take to travel to your appointment. Factor in any special conditions such as road construction, the weather, or special events that might slow down traffic (even if you are using public transportation). Plan on being out the door fifteen minutes early. Organize everything you will need, such as papers, keys, checkbook, purse or wallet, before you allow yourself to do anything else. Remember, it is more difficult to find things when you are in a panic to get out the door.

If you have a *little* time to spare, consider simply leaving early and bringing along a book or something else to occupy your time once you reach your destination. If you have a lot of time to spare, consider using a timer to remind you when to leave. You may want to buy a timer that you can pin onto your clothing so you won't run the risk of not hearing it. Don't start doing something that could be difficult to leave when it is time to go.

If you have difficulty accomplishing tasks in a timely fashion, step back and consider whether you have reasonable expectations about how long a task should take or how much can be done in one span of time. Rather than trying to "multi-task," see if you can keep yourself focused on one task at a time. Resist the urge to leave what you are doing to work on something else that comes to your attention. Most people find that they are actually more productive in the long run if one task is tackled at a time.

It is easier to talk about incorporating time-management skills than it is to implement those changes, but it is worthwhile to keep trying. Making small changes in time-management can make a big difference in your life.

The Impact of Your Depression on Friends and Family

Talking about depression

People often do not talk about their own depression, and those close to them rarely do either. It is as if there is a conspiracy of silence while everyone dances around the proverbial white elephant in the living room. People may not openly acknowledge your depression, yet it impacts everyone.

Friends and family members are sometimes completely in the dark or they may notice changes in you but not understand the cause. You may think that they know what is going on when in actuality they do not. If you put on a good front, pretending that nothing is wrong, your family and friends might not even suspect that there is a problem. You can build a wall around yourself, withdraw, and present a blank or hostile exterior to those around you. This type of behavior may lead to arguments or stony silences in your home. If this is happening, it's time to do something.

Regardless of whether your depression is well

hidden or obvious, it is helpful to break the silence. There isn't anything to be ashamed about. It may take time before you truly believe that, but eventually it will be easier to accept the fact that it's not your fault. Opening up communication is the first step in the healing process for families. You may think that other people won't understand what you're going through, but you could be surprised. Even if they don't fully understand depression, they can be supportive. Many people have difficulty discussing depression. If you feel uncomfortable about opening up to family or friends, a psychotherapist or psychiatrist may be able to help. Obtaining some basic information about depression can help the whole family.

Silence breeds misunderstanding

When depression is unrecognized or misunderstood, friends and family members react in their own individual ways. People may think that something other than depression is accounting for your behavior. A spouse or significant other may assume that you don't love them anymore, or think that you have withdrawn because you are involved with someone else. They may think that they are doing something to make you act angry, withdrawn, or sad. If you detach and isolate, they may feel abandoned, angry, sad, insecure, or unloved. In turn, they may react by withdrawing from you. They may think that you are acting this way on purpose.

Misperceptions about depression are common

Misperceptions about depression can affect the way in which people relate to you. If your loved ones believe that depression is a choice you have made and that you should be able to snap out of it, they may not be patient or supportive.

Many people erroneously believe that if you simply did something enjoyable, the depression would go away. It can be hard for them to imagine that you could still feel terrible even when things in your life seem fine. The fact is, even if the best thing in the world happened to you, depression can persist. Stressors can precipitate or worsen depression, but an episode can occur without being caused by anything. Family members may ask you about what caused your depression, assuming that something is bothering you. They may believe that you can be talked out of it. They may have a hard time understanding that the main thing bothering you is the depression itself.

The people in your life may be struggling

Everyone close to you is affected by your depression, just as surely as if you had cancer. Family members and friends may overcompensate, trying to do more for you with the hope that it will turn things around. If your depression has been severe or prolonged they might feel like they are at the end of their rope: worn down, helpless, frustrated, and uncertain about what to do. If your loved ones feel like everything they say and do is taken the wrong way, they may avoid conversation for fear of being the target of your anger. If you don't want their help and push them away without explanation, they might stop reaching out to you. Your loved ones may have no idea how to help. Their world can be turned upside down and they don't know how to fix it.

People often take on new roles when a family member has depression. A spouse may have taken over responsibility for certain things that were previously the domain of the person with depression. The afflicted person may have taken on a more dependent role while ill (as is true with most illnesses). When the depression begins to lift, people are no longer as dependent and everyone has to readjust as roles shift again.

If the people in your life are struggling with your depression or the changes that are taking place as you begin to feel better, consider including them in the treatment process. Everyone can benefit if your loved ones are given informaton about depression and if they have the opportunity to ask questions. Involving them in your therapy can give them a forum where feelings can be discussed constructively and they may have valuable insights. Therapy can help to establish healthy coping strategies, clear up misunderstandings, resolve conflicts, build trust, and enhance communication. Being able to look at things from another person's perspective generally helps everybody to achieve a stronger relationship.

Children of a depressed parent

Care should be taken so that children are not put in the position of providing emotional support for their parent. It is not healthy for children to be used as sounding boards. They need to be able to be children and have adults take care of themselves.

A child may think that they are to blame for their parent's behavioral changes. They may think that it is their responsibility to fix things, go out of their way to try to please their parent or try to provide comfort. It is important to reassure them that the problem is being addressed and that they are not the problem.

Children may try to take on the role of peacemaker when their parent is angry. Let them know that they are not responsible for making things better. Because children are frequently at the receiving end of their parent's irritability, let them know that it isn't about them, that the depression is the problem. Unfortunately, sharp or hurtful words are remembered with far more clarity than most people realize, and have the potential to hurt for years. If children have been yelled at unjustly, apologies are important. It's okay to let them know when you are feeling crabby, and then if you need some quiet time, take it. They may feel reassured to know that you're doing something to help manage your emotional state.

If there is a lot of discord between the adults in the household, it is important to shield children from arguments. Children should not be put in the middle of disagreements and parents should avoid "bad-mouthing" the other parent in front of their child. Respectful disagreement between adults is not damaging and can provide a healthy model for conflict resolution, but ongoing tension and bitter disputes adversely affect children.

Children can be given age-appropriate information to help them understand what is happening. A younger child might simply be told that their mom or dad is feeling sick, that the illness makes their parent tired or crabby or sad, and that they are seeing a doctor to help them feel better. An older child could be told that a parent is dealing with depression, a brain illness that can be treated, and then given some written information that would help them understand it better. Children should not be privy to information that belongs in the adult realm, such as suicidal thoughts or threats. Exposure to these violent thoughts can leave them feeling helpless and afraid, or they may feel responsible for the safety of their parent. Guilty feelings or a fear of abandonment may develop, which can affect a child into their adult life. Children who have had a parent commit suicide are at increased risk for eventually attempting suicide themselves.

Concern for your safety

Family and friends often worry about suicide but don't know how to talk to you about it. You may not have a clear idea of how worrisome this is or how devastating suicide is for family members. Let people know if you are having suicidal thoughts, but be careful not to use this as a way to test their love for you. Don't ask someone to keep your suicidal thoughts secret. People with depression sometimes tell themselves that everyone would be better off if they were gone, but this simply isn't true. It is important to let someone know if you are seriously considering suicide.

What Can Friends and Family Members Do to Help?

Understand that depression is an illness

Simply understanding that depression is an illness, and that the person isn't being purposefully difficult, can mean a lot. Being critical or using a "tough love" approach is no more helpful than it would be if they had some other illness, like cancer. Even though you may not truly know how they feel, you can acknowledge their pain and let them know you care. Let them know that even if you don't exactly understand depression, you know they feel terrible. Recognizing that they are ill can help them with the unwarranted burden of shame that they may feel. People with depression often worry that others will think "it's all in their head." Don't expect someone to just snap out of it and don't blame them for their illness. People don't want to feel depressed. Depression is a miserable illness, and people suffering from it may be filled with despair. They may feel like they have lost the person they were in the past. The sense of loss, fear, and anxiety that they experience can be agonizing. Let them know that you believe they can feel better again, once their depression is treated.

Treat them like a person

It is important for a person with depression to be able to maintain a sense of dignity, self-respect, and autonomy. If the depressed person is an adult, do not treat them like a child. They may be having difficulty functioning at present, but they are not oblivious to being treated differently. They will probably be extremely sensitive to shifts in the dynamics of a relationship. Most people with depression worry about being viewed as somehow different, less intelligent, abnormal, or crazy. You may want to ask them for guidance and suggestions that they think would be helpful. They need your understanding and empathy, but not sympathy. If they sense pity, they may feel worse about themselves. Let them know that you want to be helpful but that you also do not want to be intrusive. Negotiate the level of involvement that would feel respectful to them. It may feel like you are walking on a tightrope at times, but if all parties are willing to communicate openly, it's usually possible to strike some sort of balance.

Try to let them know that you don't view depression as a weakness. Be available to listen to them but don't feel like you have to give advice or have all the answers. They might simply appreciate knowing that they could tell you how they are feeling, without worrying that you are going to think you are responsible for trying to fix things for them. If they feel guilty and worry about being a burden, reassure them that "being there through thick and thin" is a part of caring for someone. Let them know how important they are to you. Remind them of times when they supported you or express your belief that, if the tables were turned, they would be there for you.

If it seems like all your efforts to reach out are rejected, you could let them know that you care and want to help but don't know how. You may want to check in periodically to see if things have changed. If they don't want your involvement, don't take it personally. Their reluctance to accept help may be a part of the depressive process or simply a reflection of their individual coping style. Remember, you can't fix it; you can only be there for them.

Try not to get pulled into arguments

Depression often causes irritability, and people may become angry without much provocation. You may feel like you are walking on eggshells, like you can't say or do anything for fear that it might be taken the wrong way. Most of the time, family members bear the brunt of this crankiness. Try not to get defensive or take it personally, and try not to retaliate if possible. If you can step back, detach yourself from the situation and try to understand what is eating at them (if anything), rather than reacting in anger—it may defuse the situation. You don't have to be a doormat, but try not to be pulled into their irritability. The anger isn't necessarily about you, but even if it is, it may be out of proportion to the trigger. People with depression don't typically enjoy being angry. Later they may realize that they overreacted and feel guilty, which reinforces their belief that they are bad. Although you are human and may not always be able to keep your cool, if you can discuss the problem calmly with them, it may help to prevent the situation from escalating. Sometimes they might not even realize that they are coming across as irritable, and it may help to tactfully remark that they seem angry and ask if something is bothering them.

Don't buy into negative thoughts

During a depressive episode, people often lose their perspective and have irrational, pessimistic thoughts. They automatically assume the worst. Even an eternal optimist can become a pessimistic curmudgeon when in the midst of a depressive episode. People develop a distorted view of the past, present, and future. Anything negative tends to get blown out of proportion; its importance in the scheme of things gets exaggerated. A negative experience can become overgeneralized in an unrealistic fashion (e.g. statements such as "If I'm no good at this then I'll never be any good at anything I try to do"). Remind them of their past successes or strengths. Later, when they do feel better, people usually look back in disbelief that they could have been thinking so negatively. For the time being, however, these negative interpretations of the world seem the most logical to them. If you can think of alternate ways of looking at things, offer those thoughts for consideration but don't feel like you have to fix everything. You can listen and be supportive but you can't possibly be your loved one's psychotherapist.

It can be extremely difficult for a person with depression to remember what it was like to feel good. Bad memories or negative thoughts are accessed more readily and it is difficult to recall good memories. A person with depression may not be able to fathom the possibility of feeling better. The all-consuming nature of depression can be compared to other intense experiences. For example, a woman in the throes of childbirth generally is not able to think of anything beyond the moment. During any intensely painful experience it can be impossible to recollect what it feels like to not be in such pain. Conversely, once a person has gotten through a difficult experience it can be hard to truly recall how bad they felt previously.

Try not to dismiss your loved one's feelings or label their thoughts as stupid or silly. That doesn't mean you have to buy into the thoughts or the hopelessness. Encourage them to try to set aside some of their worrisome thoughts for the time being and focus on what they can do to get through the day. Dwelling on problems they can't fix or control will make them feel worse. People can't be talked out of depression, but they can be encouraged and given a message of hope; it will take some time, but they can feel better. These negative thoughts and symptoms will improve as the depression is treated. Their problems won't necessarily go away, but they will be better equipped to cope with difficulties.

Add structure to the day

When a person is depressed, it can be difficult for them to decide what to do during the day. Everything can seem overwhelming. Sometimes people wander around, not knowing what to do with themselves, or stay in bed because it seems too difficult to face the day. Planning, prioritizing, and organizational skills are impaired. Adding some structure to each day can help decrease the sense of chaos that they are experiencing. Some people would not welcome, or might resent, suggestions about how to structure the day. Others might appreciate some guidance. If so, work with them on a plan.

Understand that your friend or loved one is not currently functioning at full capacity and probably can't do everything at the same level as before. This does not reflect laziness. Most people want to feel competent, but when someone has depression, they are struggling just to keep their head above water. Something that they didn't think twice about in the past can now seem like an impossible chore. If your friend or loved one has always been a "take-charge" sort of person, they may push themselves beyond their limits and feel completely overwhelmed. Friends or family members may need to take over some responsibilities for the person with depression, but rather than automatically taking over all duties, try to help them assess what they can handle at present and what they need help with. Help them set small goals but try not to pester and nag. Setting a goal and accomplishing a task can increase feelings of self-worth and a sense of competence.

Try to plan at least one small activity for the morning, afternoon, and evening. The morning task could simply be getting out of bed and showering. The afternoon activity could be a small chore, and the evening task could be a short walk. Remember, the task should be something small, something that can be accomplished. If the tasks are beyond their current capacity, they may feel overwhelmed or think of themselves as a failure. As their depression improves, they can challenge themselves with something that takes more effort.

Encourage some activities and social interaction

Your friend or loved one may need some gentle cajoling to get out of the house. They may not want to do anything, but getting out or being with other people might help them feel better, even if just briefly. Although they may not feel better immediately, the distraction of activity can help them to focus on something other than their depression. When people spend too much time alone with their thoughts, they tend to feel worse. The more a person avoids going out, the worse they imagine it will be. Eventually a person can conjure up overwhelming fear that traps them inside their own home.

Many people don't want to go out or make plans to do anything when they are depressed because they are not certain that they will feel well when the time comes. When inviting the person with depression to venture out, pick activities that aren't too intense or crowded. Situations in which a lot of small talk is required are often difficult. Consider ways to limit the amount of time you plan to be out. Let them know that they can always go home if they want to, but that you hope that they will give it a try. If they can bring themselves to do something, they often discover that the activity goes better than they imagined it would.

During depression there is an enormous tendency to withdraw and isolate, even for people who are usually quite social. Because your friend or loved one may not initiate phone calls, you may need to take the initiative to call them. They may not return calls, even if they would like to talk to you. Not returning calls can be one of the telltale signs that things are not going well. It's part of the depressive process. Keep trying and don't take it personally. This probably won't be a reciprocal relationship until their depression begins to improve.

Give them some breathing room

Although some level of activity and social interaction should be encouraged, bear in mind that the person with depression may need some time alone; some quiet, peaceful time. They may simply want some time at home with you. Too much stimulation and noise, or too many people, may leave them feeling nervous and tense. Try not to hover or watch every move they make; they may feel smothered. People without depression generally desire a mixture of social and private time, activity and rest. This kind of balance is generally good for a person with depression as well.

Provide reassurance

Offer realistic hopefulness about the likelihood for recovery with appropriate treatment; it won't happen overnight, but they can get better. Your friend or loved one may imagine the "worst case scenario" in all aspects of their life. Try to avoid telling them that they "should just stop worrying, everything will be all right" but instead offer alternate ways of looking at things. Your friend or loved one may feel very insecure or fearful, have a hard time being alone, or want you close at hand. It can be tiring to provide them with the same assurances over and over, but their neediness may be part of their illness. Their depression may have robbed them of the ability to be reassured in any sustained fashion. Like trying to bring water home in a bucket full of holes, reassurance escapes them. The bucket can be filled up over and over, but it is soon empty. It is important to keep in mind, however, that even though they may not find lasting comfort in your words, your repeated reassurances and belief that they will get better may be one of the things that helps them get through the tough times.

Suicidal thoughts

If your friend or loved one talks about suicide, it's a signal to get professional help immediately. Don't assume that the threats are "attention-seeking" behaviors, or that just because they are talking about their thoughts that they won't act on them. Depression can be so difficult to endure that people contemplate suicide as a way to escape. People often don't realize that they can feel like themselves again. They cannot imagine having to feel this way forever and death may seem like the only way to make it end. What people are generally seeking is relief, an end to the pain. They would like to feel better, but if they think that they cannot, death may seem preferable.

Some people may have no idea that what they are suffering from is depression. They know something is terribly wrong, but they have no idea about what to do or where to turn. In a state of hopelessness, they may try to commit suicide.

It might seem incomprehensible that someone could possibly think of abandoning their loved ones by committing suicide. Someone with depression might not be able to see beyond the pain of what they are experiencing, let alone think realistically about how anyone else would feel if they died. They may not be thinking rationally at this point. Their thought processes can be disorganized and they may have severely impaired problem-solving capabilities. Overwhelmed and with no way to cope, they turn to suicide.

Depression can be a huge challenge for everyone involved. It is not unusual for people to think that they are a burden to their loved ones and that everyone would be better off if they were dead. They think others would "get over" their death and then be able to get on with their lives. These beliefs are promoted by the thought distortions that come with depression.

Alcohol intoxication is a risk factor for suicide; it clouds judgment and people tend to feel more despondent and hopeless when intoxicated, leading them to take action that they normally would not. Significant stressors, such as legal or financial problems, loss of a job or a relationship, or the death of a loved one, can tip a depressed person over the edge toward suicide.

People are also at risk for suicide when they are just beginning to get better, have more energy, and can think clearly enough to actually come up with a plan to kill themselves. At this point, they may have improved enough to be able to take some action, but not enough that there is any noticeable improvement in their mood or hopelessness. If a person suddenly starts getting their affairs in order, giving away possessions, or making a flurry of calls to all the people who are close to them, it may be a signal that they are suicidal. When people have made the decision to commit suicide, they sometimes appear more calm, at ease, and energized. Because they may believe that suicide is the only way to end their suffering, making the decision can seem like a big relief to them. They need to know that they can get better. They don't need to die to change the way they're feeling. They just need some help.

To reiterate, if a person talks about suicide, seek professional help immediately. Remove firearms from the home and take any other reasonable or necessary precautions to limit easy access to potentially lethal items. You may need to closely monitor the person with depression prior to their evaluation by a professional, or call 911 if they are acutely suicidal and unwilling to be evaluated. It is not pleasant to have to resort to calling 911—and the person brought in for evaluation against their will may harbor feelings of anger and resentment for a while—but when people have recovered enough to think clearly, it is not unusual for them to feel grateful that you cared enough to risk their anger in order to keep them safe. Most people who attempt suicide are later thankful that they did not succeed.

It is also important to remember that even caring and watchful family and friends, doctors and therapists cannot always predict or prevent a suicide attempt by a person determined to end their life. If the worst happens and your loved one takes their life, seek help and support for yourself. Suicide of a loved one is one of the most painful, traumatic, and unfathomable experiences that people have to endure. It isn't your fault. If possible, try to attend a support group. You aren't alone.

Obtaining professional help

A person with depression may need some support in order to seek help. They may not even recognize that they have depression. If you can express the reasons why you are concerned, in a compassionate, nonjudgmental manner, it may help them to identify that there really is a problem. They may feel a sense of shame and resist going in for treatment, but it's worthwhile to keep encouraging them to do so. The decision whether to seek treatment or not is ultimately in their hands (unless they are acutely suicidal or dangerous to others), but words of encouragement can make all the difference. Let them know that you care about them, no matter what, that they are important to you and that you want them to feel better. If you have had depression and are now better, share that with them. That information may provide hope and make it easier for them to discuss their problem. Let them know that seeking help is a sign of strength, not a sign of weakness.

People with depression can feel immobilized and may not know how or where to get help. They might need assistance with arranging an appointment, though most doctors' offices will require that they call to schedule the appointment themselves. It is often important for the doctor to gather some preliminary information directly from the person with depression. If someone is actively involved in scheduling their own appointment, they may also be more likely to follow through with it.

Family members sometimes hope that if they schedule an appointment without the depressed person's knowledge and somehow get them to the office, things will work out. However, using coercion or bringing someone in under duress rarely works well. People who are "surprised" with an appointment often become angry and refuse to participate in the session. Very little is accomplished and they may be even less inclined to seek help in the future. However, as previously noted, the exception to this general principle is the situation in which a person is acutely suicidal and not willing to pursue treatment voluntarily.

Although there are good reasons to require that someone personally schedule their own appointment, having to make the call can present an obstacle. You may need to walk them through the process.

If your friend or loved one has a few good days, it can be tempting to think that things are beginning to turn around. Keep in mind that they may have an up and down course, with some days better than others. Good days are encouraging, but a few good days don't necessarily mean the depression is gone. If there are still bad days, they are likely still suffering from depression and should be encouraged to seek treatment.

If necessary, help them follow their treatment program

Many people do not need reminders about taking their medication and making appointments with their doctor, but some people have a hard time remembering to do these things. If your friend or loved one seems to need help, talk about it. They might simply need a reminder to take their medicine, help with organizing medication in a weekly dispenser, or you may need to provide more direct supervision. If they are having problems with side effects or seem to be doing worse, you may need to encourage them to call their doctor. Ask to be included in some of their appointments; your loved one may not automatically invite you and the doctor cannot communicate with you directly unless they are given written permission.

If your friend or family member has been encouraged to get some exercise, offer to take a walk with them. You may feel frustrated if their recovery progress is slow, but try not to nag. If they are not eating, try to help them think of some palatable foods or supplemental shakes. If they eat too much to try to feel better, don't make disparaging comments about their eating habits or weight. Instead, try to make some healthy food choices available and leave it at that.

Keep your eyes open but don't discount or overscrutinize their moods

Once a person recovers from depression, they often worry that everything they say and do is under scrutiny, that they are under a microscope. People want to be taken at face value and not have their moods questioned or feelings discounted. Family members naturally may be watchful for mood changes, for fear that the depression might come back and, in actuality, may recognize changes even before the person with depression does. Some negotiation may need to take place so that the concerned family member has permission to respectfully bring up their concerns, without fear that the person who has recovered will get defensive and angry.

It is important to understand that people who have had depression may not recognize signs that it is returning. They may be so used to coping with depression by continuing to put one foot in front of the other that they do not identify the early signs. It is also fairly normal for people to attribute their symptoms to outside stressors without realizing that those stresses may have triggered an actual depressive episode. People dread the thought of dipping back down into depression and do not want to even think about the possibility that it might have returned.

Family members also need to recognize that treatment for depression doesn't wipe out all emotions. A goal in treating depression is a return to a normal range of feelings that are proportional and appropriate to the context of a person's life. People who have recovered from depression will be able to experience happiness again, but they will also still feel anger, anxiety, and sadness. Be careful not to attribute every uncomfortable emotion to depression. Once a person has recovered from depression, they are not immune to occasional crankiness; even people without depression can have a bad day. One of the last things a person who has recovered from depression wants to hear is the question "Have you been taking your medication?" It is not fair to use this question in an angry, accusatory fashion. Only ask this question if you truly are worried and then consider first prefacing it with some of your concerns or observations.

Take care of yourself

Depression takes a toll on everyone in the family and can be just as difficult to deal with as any other significant illness. It is very important for family members to take care of themselves, or they also risk burnout and depression. This point can't be overemphasized. Dealing with depression can become overwhelming and isolating for everyone involved. Try to maintain your own routine and normal activities as much as possible.

You may worry that things will never change, especially if you have no idea about what is happening with your loved one's treatment plan. At times you may feel exasperated, angry, worn down, lonely, apprehensive about the future, sad, or helpless. This is when it is especially important to consider asking to be included in some sessions with the doctor in order to be better informed about what is going on and to provide your insight about progress. Having everyone on the same page, with a clear idea about what is going on, can be invaluable. Even when a person is following their treatment plan to the letter, they may not have the desired response. Ask for help if you need it. If you are struggling, consider seeing a therapist yourself rather than trying to shoulder the stress all alone.

Learning more about depression by reading books can help you feel less powerless and confused. Support groups can also be a valuable resource. Attending a support group for friends and family members can help you feel less alone, and being exposed to other people's experiences may give you insights about your own situation.

Concluding Remarks

Learning more about depression

Knowing more about depression can help you take better care of yourself and can be the key to freeing yourself from the stigma of the illness. Reading books and talking with other people can be invaluable. There are a number of good books about depression; I recommend that you read several of them. Find books with the level of complexity that suits your purposes. Authors may express different opinions. By reading different books, you will come away with a more balanced understanding of the pertinent issues. Look for rounded approaches. Be cautious of books or treatment programs that proclaim they offer "the solution" for depression. Internet sites from professional organizations or other reliable sources can be useful (note the emphasis on reliable—the Internet also affords ample opportunity for misinformation). Community and national support groups also provide valuable information.

What you can do for other people once you feel better

Simply stated, pass the word. While it may be prudent to be careful about disclosing information about depression in certain situations, such as in a work setting, on a personal level you may recognize symptoms in other people and be able to help someone else because of your experience. Depression often goes untreated simply because it is unrecognized. People also often have an easier time acknowledging depression if they are aware that others have it as well. Knowing that someone else has experienced similar feelings and symptoms can make all the difference to someone suffering from depression. This knowledge helps reduce unwarranted feelings of shame and provides hope that things can get better, which in turn may increase the likelihood that someone will consider being evaluated for depression. There is a wonderful ripple effect after a person has been treated, feels better, and then shares that information. If you recognize the symptoms of depression in someone close to you, your insights and experience can be invaluable to them. A gentle nudge can be a marvelous gift.

Recommended Reading

Ainsworth, Patricia, M.D. 2000. *Understanding Depression*. Jackson: University Press of Mississippi.

DePaulo, J. Raymond, Jr., M.D., and Leslie Alan Horvitz. 2002. *Understanding Depression*. Hoboken, N.J.: John Wiley & Sons.

Gilbert, Paul. 2001. *Overcoming Depression*. New York: Oxford University Press.

Medina, John, Ph.D. 1998. *Depression: How it Happens, How it's Healed*. Hong Kong: New Harbinger Publications.

Papolos, Demitri, M.D., and Janice Papolos. 1997. *Overcoming Depression*. New York: HarperCollins.

Rosen, Laura Epstein, Ph.D., and Xavier Francisco Amador, Ph.D. 1997. *When Someone You Love Is Depressed*. New York: Simon & Schuster, Inc.

Resources

American Psychiatric Association
1400 K St. N.W.
Washington, DC 20005
(202) 682-6850
Web Site: www.psych.org

American Psychological Association
750 First St. N.E.
Washington, DC 20002-4242
(800) 374-2721
(202) 336-5510
TDD/TTY: (202) 336-6123
Web Site: www.apa.org

National Institute of Mental Health (NIMH)
Public Inquiries
6001 Executive Blvd., Room 8184, MSC 9663
Bethesda, MD 20892-9663
(301) 443-4513
TTY: (301) 443-8431
Fax: (301) 443-4279
Web Site: www.nimh.nih.gov

Depression Awareness, Recognition and Treatment (D/ART)
National Institute of Mental Health
5600 Fishers Lane
Rockville, MD 20857
(800) 421-4211

National Alliance for the Mentally Ill (NAMI)
2107 Wilson Blvd., Suite 300
Arlington, VA 22201
(703) 524-7600
(800) 950-NAMI (6264)
Fax: (703) 524-9094
Web Site: www.nami.org

National Mental Health Association
1021 Prince Street
Alexandria, VA 22314-2971
(703) 684-7722
Information Line (800) 969-NMHA (6642)
Fax: (703) 684-5968
Web Site: www.nmha.org

National Foundation for Depressive Illness
P.O. Box 2257
New York, NY 10116
(212) 268-4260 or (800) 239-1265
Fax: (212) 268-4434

Depression and Bipolar Support Alliance
730 North Franklin Street, Suite 501
Chicago, IL 60610-7224
(800) 826-3632
(312) 642-0049
Fax: (312) 642-7243
Web Site: www.DBSAlliance.org

Suicide Awareness Voices of Education (SA/VE)
7317 Cahill Road, Suite 207
Minneapolis, MN 55439-0507
(952) 946-7998 or 1-888-511-SAVE
Web Site: www.save.org

Acknowledgments

I am indebted to Matthew Collins for his thoughtful insights, suggestions, and reviews of this manuscript. Many thanks to Nora Collins, Lynne Dolan and Dr. Peggy Baker for their constructive commentary and encouragement. Special thanks go to the many people who have provided invaluable support, including Jane Schultz, R.N.—wonderful nurse, kindred spirit, dear friend. Jane Thompson, MSW, LICSW, BCD—ever irreverent friend with good shoes and a lot of letters after her name. Lou Bartholome, LP—terrific colleague and therapist. Debbra Ford, Psy.D.—smart, funny friend who plays a mean piano and is a darn good therapist. And Cheryl Karpen, my friend since childhood, with thanks for the strawberries, mud, and inspiration.

Lesli N. Kramer, M.D., is a graduate of the University of Minnesota Medical School. After completing her internship at the Hennepin County Medical Center in Minneapolis, MN, and her psychiatry residency at the University of Minnesota Medical School, she practiced psychiatry in a large multi-specialty group practice for ten years prior to entering her private practice in Eden Prairie, MN.

To order additional copies of *Recovering from Depression:*

Web: www.itascabooks.com

Phone: 1-800-901-3480

Fax: Copy and fill out the form below with credit card information. Fax to 651-603-9263.

Mail: Copy and fill out the form below. Mail with check or credit card information to:

Syren Book Company
C/O BookMobile
2402 University Avenue West
Saint Paul, Minnesota 55114

Order Form

Copies	Title / Author	Price	Totals	
	***Recovering from Depression* / Kramer**	$16.95	$	
	Subtotal		$	
	7% sales tax (MN only)		$	
	Shipping and handling, first copy		$	4.00
	Shipping and handling, ___ add'l copies @$1.00 ea.		$	
	TOTAL TO REMIT		$	

Payment Information:

__ Check Enclosed __ Visa/Mastercard		
Card number:	Expiration date:	
Name on card:		
Billing address:		
City:	State:	Zip:
Signature :	Date:	

Shipping Information:

__ Same as billing address __ Other (enter below)		
Name:		
Address:		
City:	State:	Zip: